Wome...
Weight Loss Tamasha

Praise for Rujuta's debut book
Don't Lose Your Mind, Lose Your Weight

When did you last read a diet book by an Indian writer that was readable, funny, well-organised, sensible and persuasive, all at the same time? Told you both the rules and how to cheat intelligently, if you slipped up?

— **Anjali Puri, Outlook**

Page by page, chapter by chapter Rujuta explains how practically everything we have accepted as the gospel truth when it comes to dieting is wrong ... And what works is the way Rujuta gets her point across. Totally candid, down to earth, bindaas ... This is a book grounded in a philosophy of life. A confluence as it were of all that Rujuta has learned (and is still learning) from her study of yoga, ayurveda, sports science and nutrition.

–**Rashmi Bansal**

So, I ate every couple of hours. I drank intimidating quantities of water (Rujuta recommends five litres, though I never really accomplished that). I tried to follow the meal plan. Rujuta said I'd feel results immediately. I hate to sound like one of those nauseatingly ecstatic TV advertisements, but she was right. I was so cheerful, energetic and bouncy that my friends found me positively irritating.

–**Shonali Muthalaly, Hindu**

At the end of two months — with a great many transgressions — I lost almost six kilos. I am back to wearing long-forgotten pairs of jeans. My diet is now a conversation topic, and I hold forth on it like a veteran.
– Bisakha De Sarkar, Telegraph

The good thing about Diwekar is that she connects immediately with her talk about simple foods and reaching out for what one can afford versus unattainable goals and expensive food.
– Sulekha Nair, Financial Express

'Not just a delightful read but is full of handy solutions on ... how to lose weight without giving up your favourite food.'
–DNA

'[Is] fast winning a sisterhood of previously hungry women sick of their unsuccessful diets.'
–Femina

'A book that challenges you to eat to lose weight, that too, without excluding carbs... Inspiring.'
– New Woman

'The new diet bible.'
– People

WOMEN
&THE
WEIGHT
LOSS
TAMASHA

Rujuta Diwekar

westland

westland ltd

Venkat Towers, 165, P.H. Road, Maduravoyal, Chennai 600 095

No.38/10 (New No.5), Raghava Nagar, New Timber Yard Layout, Bangalore 560 026

Survey No. A-9, II Floor, Moula Ali Industrial Area, Moula Ali, Hyderabad 500 040

23/181, Anand Nagar, Nehru Road, Santacruz East, Mumbai 400 055

47, Brij Mohan Road, Daryaganj, New Delhi 110 002

First published by westland ltd 2010

ISBN 978-93-80658-33-9

Typeset in Minion Pro by Ram Das Lal

Printed at Thomson Press (I) Ltd.

*A portion of the proceeds from the sale of this book go to Nirantar Trust.
We thank you for supporting this intiative with your purchase.*

For you again, Bebo ...
For making eating fashionable

Contents

A Personal Note From Kareena Kapoor

Kareena Kapoor

"oh God! I'm so busy today, I have no time to eat". The fastest selling excuse, easy to say and believe. Ever thought, "I hardly ate anything today. I better feel and look thin..." Or, I am hardly eating. Why am I not losing weight?" Now my response to that is what my darling Rujuta Diwekar has taught me: "PLEASE EAT" or you are not going to loose weight.

Now, as an actress who works 18-20 hours a day, under gruelling circumstances (its -7°C sometimes, other times 50°c), shooting all night, playing and feeling a range of emotions - some days I have to cry a lot, and sometimes despite having my periods. I have to dance in the rain, trying to look beautiful and above all, trying to look and stay slim. But like I said come hail or storm, every 2-3 hours, my stomach makes a loud call of hunger, and like a good girl I attend to it. Now I am sure all the women reading this book probably don't have to dance in the rain, but definately have so many demands

→

On their time, its not that difficult, though, to slip in a slice of cheese, some peanuts or an apple in your handbag. Believe me, its all about the habit. It takes a week to cultivate a habit of stopping whatever you're doing for just two minutes to grab a bite. I wouldn't give up my profession no matter what, its the most important thing in my life, but looking after my health and eating habits is a non-negotiable aspect of my life and its what keeps me going.

A very important aspect of us women are our ever changing hormones that lead to mood swings, acne, bloating and hair fall... We deal with a lot don't we?? Pregnancy cravings? oh! its all a part of it my lovely ladies. My advice is no need to scream "PANIC" when all these things happen. Just take out the time to EAT RIGHT. The day I come back from a long flight, I am extremely bloated, my hands and feet are swollen because of water retention, jet lag, lack of sleep and air pressure. But like rujuta says, lots of water and a home remedy of

Kareena Kapoor

ghar Ka Khana - Some light dal, sabzi, and rice - and immediately restarting my two-Lovely diet, and the next day I instantly see the difference.

Women, if may say so, have an inherent ability to be beautiful. We just need to feel beautiful, and to feel gorgeous, remember, you have to eat your way to health, fitness and ultimately, "WEIGHTLOSS". What would I have done if I hadn't met and learned this from Rujuta? I am proud to eat and eat a lot, despite being so busy.... It is the happiest feeling waiting for my next meal. It might not be bhajiyas and Vada Pav but who wants all that if I look like this and stay fit and healthy?

As I write this I am in Switzerland, enjoying the ripe fruits, berries and the yummy cheese, the fresh milk, and the avocado and aubergine sandwich in my hotel. Awesome! And I don't see myself putting on weight.... In fact, I see myself, lovely ladies, "GLOWING"!

→

Is it the berries, is it Switzerland or was it the apple pie and vanilla Ice-Cream I had last night? Oops, Sorry RUJUTA! ☺

Much Love
To all,
Kareena Kapoor

Introduction

It was almost dark by the time we reached Demul, a village high above the Spiti river. As Tshering urged our car for the final climb, we looked up at the ridge and, silhouetted against the crimson sky, were women, heads and noses covered, backs erect, riding drunk men on handsome horses. I was sure I was hallucinating, blaming it on the altitude (4300m) and my tired body (we had been forced to walk an extra thirty kilometres after our four-day trek). I looked at GP and his keen eyes mirrored the same feelings.

So it was real, then. The annual horse race had just gotten over. The men had raced their horses on the ridge and around the Baleri top for good weather and good crop. Now the women were riding the drunken men back home. I had heard GP making some noises about Spiti being a genderless society, but I was not prepared for this display of stree shakti. Coming from urban/mainland India, this concept was as real as the Yeti to me.

As I struggled to come to terms with this unabashed display, another one was being played out for me in the kitchen of our homestay. The man of the house was busy making aloo momos for us while the woman wiped the plates clean, baby-talking to her three-month-old granddaughter and talking to us in a dialect we had never heard before. Strangely, she communicated. Communicated what I needed to learn: the power over leading one's life doesn't have to dilute femininity in any way.

This then forms the theme of this book: that mindless compliance should be questioned and if found baseless, let go off. Whether it's some ideal weight or size, rituals or societal norms or role-play of a four-in-one — mother, wife, daughter (in-law) and 'career-woman'.

Why this book?

I wrote my first book because I got an offer to write, yes, but also because I felt that there was too much misinformation about weight loss floating around. Post the book, my inbox has been flooded with more horror stories (from a twenty-three-year-old who surgically got her stomach strapped to control her appetite, to a devastated seventeen-year-old who got liposuction as her eighteenth birthday gift, and the most horrific one being of a thirty-six-year-old wanting to commit suicide because she couldn't lose the last five kilos even after starving herself for the last forty-two days) than I can handle and a lot of them are from women.

Honestly, I think eating right, working out, sleeping on time, cultivating healthy relationships — the basic stuff — should be part of our school curriculum, that way at least we will have some basic understanding about our bodies, keeping it fit, healthy and leading a fulfilling life.

I wrote this book because women I met, interacted and worked with often displayed a kind of helplessness. A helplessness over their lives, over the roles they had confined themselves to, the dreams and goals that they had buried long ago, over their hormones, over their body weight and even over the size of their jeans.

Women, however, are far from helpless; they are helpful, resourceful, compassionate, warm, loving and focused individuals. In my office, a married man almost never walks in alone for his appointment, he is always accompanied by his wife or daughter-in-law. They come to support him in his efforts to get fitter, leaner, stronger, healthier, and are willing to go all the way to ensure that no hurdles come in the way of his fitness. Married women, however, come alone; they plead helplessness over the ways of cooking and eating in the family, cite school timings or preferred meal timings when asked to make time to workout or advance dinner times. When it comes to the men or children in the family, their health, fitness and wellness, the women will change everything: meal timings, cooking styles, bedtimes, workouts, etc. When it comes to using the exact same resources for themselves, they can't, the same drivers of change are helpless.

In a country like ours, where goddesses are worshipped as shakti, loosely translated as strength or power, this helplessness is out of sync with our belief system, our history of Razia Sultan, Rani Laxmibai and even our current political and corporate culture scene with women occupying positions of power at almost all levels. Even as I say this, a part of me says – Ya, in a country like ours, where bahus are decorated and burnt, foetuses dropped and daughters murdered or married, all for the family's imagined honour or status, what power do we really have over our body weight, much less our life? Through the book you will find me struggling to stick to the point of our discussion — weight loss, fitness, wellness. Invariably while making an important point related to food, exercise, sleep or relationships, I digress into our position in the household, society, community, country and in the world at large. I do strongly believe that one of the main reasons why we allow our health, dreams, ambitions and our persona to take a backseat as we go from being little girls to married women, mothers to grandmothers, is because we take the set roles at every stage much more seriously than ourselves. For true health, fitness and well-being to come to every woman, she has to go beyond (challenge) the social convention of what is acceptable and therefore beautiful at every stage of her life. A woman with unrealised potential is unhappy, frustrated and unsettled, no matter what her marital status, body weight or waist-size.

I have written this book exactly like the way my conversations shape up with my women clients. We talk of everything under the sun: mother-in-law, father-in-law, visiting sister-in-law, projects in school, CL in office, maid troubles, traffic on the roads, break-ups, make-ups, latest fashion, molestation at train stations, and through all this we decide the meal plan for the next two weeks. So we spill the beans, cry buckets, vent anger, laugh with our heads thrown back and figure ways of when, how and whether it's worth zipping our mouths at all (or is it time to open it wide and start eating).

Regarding the name, well isn't the term '*weight loss*' worthy of a title? I mean we talk about it the most, don't we? So even though it's one of the many 'components' of the tamasha, it gets prominence in our conscious mind.

A recap of the four principles
of eating right....

Principle 1: Eat something within the first ten-fifteen minutes of getting up. Tea/coffee should not be the first thing you have when you wake up. These stimulants will increase the blood pressure, heart rate, breathing rate and only end up stressing the body. In turn, the body will respond by hampering fat burning. On the other hand, if you eat something within the first fifteen minutes of getting up, blood sugar and energy levels increase, leading to an increase in metabolic rate and fat burning, and a decrease in acidity and bloating. You're less likely to overeat later and your blood sugars remain stable through the day. Basically, there's less chance of getting fat.

Principle 2: Eat every two hours. When you eat every two hours, your meals are more likely to be small. And when our body gets a small amount of calories at one time, they're utilised better and not stored as fat (because the body feels reassured with a regular intake of calories and nutrients), which means a flatter stomach. Also, you'll depend less on stimulants during the day.

Principle 3: Eat more when you're active and less when you are not. Your body's requirements change depending on your activity (mental or physical) levels, hormonal changes, etc. Now, as you follow Principles 1 and 2, you'll get more in touch with the hunger signals your body is sending and when you feel like the need to eat more, do so. Eating more food when you're more active will make your body an efficient calorie burner, which will increase the metabolic rate of your body. This will make you stay energetic through the day and will help you lose fat more effectively.

Principle 4: Finish your last meal at least two hours prior to sleeping. An extension of Principle 3 — eat less post sunset and as your activities wind down. This way, most of your food is digested before you go to sleep, which will lead to a sound sleep, and leaves your body free to do its repair work.

...And the five basic rules to increase nutrient intake

1. Eat food that is prepared fresh, and eat it within three hours of cooking.
2. The smaller the number of people food is prepared for, the better its nutrient value.
3. Eat your vegetables and fruits whole; don't cut them or mash them into a juice.
4. Remain loyal to your genes: eat what you have been eating since childhood.
5. Eat what is in season. For example, mango in summer.

Chapter plan

The crux of the book are its *four strategies* of well-being which deal with our food, workout, sleep and relationships. In fact, the entire book is almost like building up my case to underline the importance and relevance of the four strategies of well-being. It goes beyond the four principles of eating right, the reason being that a woman's life is affected and gets affected by much more than food or what she eats or doesn't. When a little girl gets her first period, the last thing she is thinking is — let me eat right. She is trying to grapple with the reality of her period and that it's going to be a part of her life for the next twenty-thirty years. At this time it's her relationship with her parents (and more specifically her mother), that determines whether or not she will make a smooth transition into teenage and tweens. This forms the chapter on **puberty**.

Getting **married**, choosing to **stay single** or wanting to live-in brings a woman to another challenging phase where not just her hormones but even societal and her own expectations take a toll on her health. Marriage or a committed relationship means garam, tazaa ghar ka khana for a man, and arranging for it for a woman. She has to learn to be and stay important in her own eyes to ensure that creeping obesity doesn't set in post marriage.

Pregnancy and motherhood is exhilarating in as many ways as it is draining. Looking after a baby and being completely responsible for her food, health and well-being can get so time and energy-consuming that it's not unusual for women to forget that they even exist. She becomes invisible to herself, to her own needs to sleep or eat on time, and while this is fine for a month or two, if this becomes a pattern then the mother actually stands to harm her own baby. After all, without adequate rest, food, strength and support from family, it's almost impossible to look after a baby well. This is the one time where a woman owes herself much more responsible behaviour and good rest (sleep) than she believes.

Menopause is a totally different ball game, in many ways similar to the first period and yet with a completely different perspective. It's like a woman's life comes full-circle, the roles that she assumed purely out of biology no longer seem relevant. In many ways it's the triumph of a woman's real self over her lower self or what she has come to become.

To find out how to tweak your food according to the phase of life you are in, you will need to read about all these phases and then the Four Strategies chapter in the end. This will give you a good understanding of how your nutrient and other requirements change according to every phase of your life and whether you need to review your expectations from yourself and your body. It will help you identify if your need to lose weight is driven by a mindless compliance to the social understanding of 'beauty' — which is 'thin and fair' — or is it driven by a strong urge or responsibility towards your body, to make it fitter, stronger, leaner.

After the four stages of a woman's life (I call it four stages because it changes us hormonally and in our appearance, body weight too), I write about the curses we bring upon ourselves. Curses here is not a negative, but our body's way of bringing our attention to ourselves, her ever-forgiving and supportive nature of providing us with endless opportunities to correct our wrong-doing. **Hypothyroid** and **PCOD** get written about in detail because, when it comes to these two, I see too much helplessness again. 'I am a hopeless, defeated case, I have PCOD and I am devastated', or a similar sounding, 'I will remain fat because I have hypothyroid'. Honestly, our hormones haven't cursed us to stay fat, nor have their imbalances. Our complete lack of education about our hormones, the way they work, their function and how our food, exercise, sleep and relationships affect them has doomed us. Whether or not you have hypothyroid or PCOD, this chapter will give you much needed information about the workings of your body and will demystify the thyroid, menstrual cycle and PCOD forever (I hope). But beware, post the chapter you will not be able to blame your hormones for your troubles, including body weight or acne. I have also covered diabetes, joint problems, menstrual cramps and constipation, but not in as much detail as hypothyroid and PCOD. The reason being that most of us understand that when we get careless with our lifestyle we gain body fat and this can make us susceptible to constipation, diabetes or low back pain. But we don't seem to apply that logic with hypothyroid or PCOD.

The book ends with a comprehensive look at the four strategies of well-being, and seriously, if you have time to read only one chapter, this is the one. I hope you will enjoy reading them and that it will help you understand that life is not about losing five kilos in fifteen days. It's about pursuing our passions, making time to eat, workout, sleep, enjoying our relationships, learning to put ourselves first and, well, (cliché, cliché) enjoying the journey.

Components of the book

Real life examples of my women clients (names changed where necessary) are the anchor on which the entire book rests. Most of the chapters start with one, which typifies the struggles women face at any given phase of their life. It provides the framework to discuss how hormonally, nutritionally and emotionally our requirements alter with each phase and what changes we can make to tackle them.

Boxes have been used throughout the book to talk about anything and everything related to the topic under discussion, without breaking the flow.

Practical *strategies* for nutrition, exercise, sleep and relationships are provided for all phases specifically, apart from the in-depth review in Chapter 7.

I have also provided *actual diet recalls,* along with the corresponding evaluation and suggested modifications of women (my clients, with some names changed) in various professions, pertinent to each phase and disorder, which kind of wraps up all we have learnt in a chapter. Use the diet recall and analysis examples exactly as they are meant to be: learning tools. Use them to understand how to evaluate and modify your current eating habits while applying all that you have learnt about the specific phase or condition in that chapter. Don't blindly change your eating habits according to one of the recalls; instead spend time and effort into planning your own, keeping in mind your current lifestyle and challenges. It's really not that difficult. To further your understanding and practice of using recalls as a learning tool, I have put in a few extra in the Appendix. Have fun going through them and coming up with your own plan, but remember recalls in the book are indicators, and meal plans are suggestive, not laws.

The *Appendices* include some very interesting information on how Indian breakfasts compare to the muesli/cereal-milk combo, the effect of various nutrition deficiencies on our body, short-term and long-term effects of 'low-calorie' diets and some more real life diet analysis. I think you will find the appendices really useful to do a quick check or assessment of your current eating habits.

Another thing: old habits die hard, so to explain the workings of nutrients, hormones, enzymes, etc. (processes so complex even modern nutrition science is yet to unravel them completely), I draw analogies with things completely unrelated — cars, politics, in-laws, etc. This in no way is meant to belittle the complexities of the workings of the human body, but to make it easy for us to gain understanding of the bigger picture.

The 'take away'
The feelings of inadequacy that we have bought into stare us in our faces when we want to quickly lose weight for

a wedding, tuck our tummy in for a photograph, starve to flaunt a small paunch for that evening party, wear a corset to fit into a smaller size, over-exercise to punish ourselves from late-night bingeing. Isn't it time to end the weight loss tamasha? Isn't it high time we woke up to the many miracles of the workings of our body, her ever-loving and giving nature, and took notice of the fact that we are beautiful exactly the way we are. Not a size smaller or a few kilos less; time to celebrate our body, our femininity, our divinity…

Happy reading.

Rujuta Diwekar
Mumbai, November 2010

1

The Tamasha

Speak to any health professional in the country and they will tell you that men respond better to treatment than women, be it diabetes, malaria, weight loss or simply a pedicure. As women, we're guilty of supporting our men (father, brother, husband, son, father-in-law, son-in-law, brother-in-law) much more than we support ourselves or other women. The roots could be in the very fabric of our country, culture, tradition, religion whatever, but we don't quite treat ourselves right or as equals. The most basic way in which we treat ourselves badly, is by denying ourselves the food we love, at the time we love and in quantities we love, and then of course to make things worse, we go about our life believing that our body owes it to us to stay toned, fit, lean and thin. Which is why this chapter even exists in this book, because we have bought into the tamasha, putting our health, body, nutrients, sleep, relationships and life itself at stake. When you read on, I want you to ask yourself if you identify with the behaviour patterns cited in the chapter, because I want you to give up thinking about your body as an object which deserves shame/criticism/ something to be depressed over if it doesn't fit into some mould. I would actually sum it up with just two words — criticism kills. But if I had to write down reasons why women have such a hard time losing weight or why we behave so similar to the moon, reducing and gaining size every fortnight, here they are:

Always criticising your body
Real life example

Sarita walked in, looking fab in a black T-shirt and jeans, and got into an animated chat with Tejal, my nutritionist. They settled down in their chairs and began our usual exercise — discussing her diet recall and figuring out what went right, what went wrong, what needed to be changed and what would stay for the next two weeks. I had been listening to this conversation from my seat where I was writing some answers for an interview. Finally done, I walked out.

'Wow, Sarita, you look great!'

'Please! You always say that and you are the only one who says it.'

'Why? I'm sure Tejal told you the same thing as well.'

'Of course I did. You're really looking gorgeous, Sarita.'

'In fact, Sarita, you're looking so good, I'm going to make you some masala chai.'

'That's my weakness: I can never say no to masala chai. But, you know, I'm no longer waking up to chai in the morning; I eat a banana and actually feel good. I really never thought bananas would make me feel good! It's not so bad, not waking up to chai. But I'm still doing three cups, and am not able to cut it down.'

'Oh, come on, stop being harsh on yourself. You've cut down from eight to three cups, I think that's REALLY good, that's less than half your intake, ma'am.'

'Ya, but sometimes I do four, you know. Like today, you've asked me if I want chai. Now this will be my fourth cup and I don't have the willpower to say no.'

'Arrey, you come from a family of teachers or what?'

'Yes, my mom's one. Why?'

'Because you're so critical of your progress! You're just being nice to me by not refusing my offer to make chai; it's not that you lack willpower. You didn't exactly walk in begging for ek pyali chai, and you have cut down from eight cups of chai to three, and yet you are bothered that you have not been able to cut down on that one cup.'

'But my diet allows me only two cups.'

'Listen, it's okay. Your meal plan is a guideline, not a law that you cannot break. And you need to understand the logic behind cutting down on chai: it's to not suppress or kill appetite with a stimulant. And I think you're very much getting there, it's only been a month, come on!' I was patting her on her back.

'You really think I'm doing well?'

'Of course! I would never lie to you. I would think you are doing well even if you were down to six-seven cups from eight; every step in the right direction counts. Hello! What happened? The chai is so bad or what?'

Sarita was weeping, tears rolling down all the way to her chin. 'Nooo,' she shook her head; she was smiling through her tears, but she looked genuinely troubled. 'You know, just this morning, my husband complimented me on how good I was looking. He felt my stomach had gone down, my face was looking slimmer and my thighs were looking toned…'

'How cruel,' I joked.

'Please, I am already feeling bad. You know what I said to him?'

'No, but I can guess. You asked him to shut up.'

'No, worse. I gave him a big lecture on how he lacks integrity, how he just says things without meaning them, how I don't need his sympathy, and so what if I am fat, I am brilliant at what I do and how it's only a matter of time before I get thin so he should just stop giving me this crap.'

'Oh! Poor girl. I am so sorry. What did he say?'

'What could he say? He tried telling me that he really *could* see a difference, so I really lost it. I told him it's his fault that I'm fat, that he should have told me that I've been getting fatter. I've gained fifteen kilos in two years of being married, and this man said nothing!'

'You mean nothing critical?'

She stared at me with eyes that looked deadlier than a nuclear missile.

'You are very angry, na? He said some brilliant things to you this morning and you just resisted them with all your might. My guess is that you are only receptive to criticism — you know how to respond to it. But you are clueless about how to deal with appreciation, much less compliments.'

'You think so?'

'Absolutely. I told you that you were looking great, and Tejal said the same thing less than fifteen minutes ago, and your husband said it in the morning! Think about it.'

'Ya, actually even my team in office asked me if I was doing something because they said my face was looking better.'

'There you go. Then why are you having such a hard time accepting it?'

'Actually, it's the chai. If I don't follow my diet to perfection, I feel like I'm not doing it any justice and I'm not going to get anywhere....'

'Look Sarita, Tejal is not judging you for having a couple more cups of chai than your diet requires. It's not what Tejal thinks, it's what you think about yourself. You're judging yourself a bit too harshly. You haven't acknowledged how far you have come; your focus stays on how far you still have to go. It's a journey ya, it's not about getting to some place and getting to that place in less than four weeks or whatever. Seven-eight years of being an editor, seven-eight years of eight cups a day, and less than four weeks to overcome that habit and come down to three-four cups. Brilliant! Aren't you impressed with yourself? So, now Sarita, let's do it again.'

'What?'

'The compliment bit.' I went into rewind mode and did an action replay, walking back to my office, opening my door, looking at her and saying, 'Wow! You look great!'

This time, Sarita said, 'Thanks. I have been feeling great too....'

'Want a masala chai?'

'Yes!'

Overcome the feeling of inadequacy, accept love and appreciate your efforts

Like Sarita, most of us have to make the space in our head and heart to accept love and appreciation. On the one hand we strive for it, and on the other, we attack it if it crosses our path, or we are so indifferent to it that it rubs people the wrong way. Sarita had been married only two years and her husband still had the courage to compliment her. When women are married for longer, they almost train their husbands into submission. By that I mean they usually scold their husbands so much for saying nice things that they soon learn not to say much on this 'sensitive' topic. Women appear angry with their husbands, but they are usually just very angry with themselves. Very angry for not doing something to perfection, whatever that means. No matter what they do or what they achieve, they feel inadequate. **It's this feeling of inadequacy that we need to overcome, not our body weight.**

The roots of this can be traced to the Indian way of bringing up children, specially relevant if you belong to the middle class. Our parents are so scared of 'spoiling' us, they totally avoid saying things like well done/congrats/ keep it up, etc. If you score ninety-eight on hundred, your mom is more likely to check the paper and scold you for the 'silly mistakes' that cost you the two marks, than give you a hug and exclaim, 'Ninety-eight!!' Or if you came first on Sports Day, it's met with an indifferent 'Huh' at home. It's not that our parents didn't feel happy or proud, they were just at a loss to express it without chadhaoing us, so to keep us grounded they chose to say nothing, or worse, point at 'areas of improvement'. There is a paranoia that if the child (especially the girl child) is praised, then she may become complacent and fail to strive for perfection. Or that if the girl is to be married anyway, then why 'spoil' her with these compliments;

who knows what kind of house she will be married into and whether her talents will be nurtured there?

I grew up in a progressive family and we were just two girls. Nothing that my sister and I did or didn't do was based on our gender. But in my extended family, wherever there were boys and girls in the same family, the distinction was clear. The boys would change the tube light and the girls would do the dishes. At big family functions, the men ate first (irrespective of age, qualifications, achievements, merits-demerits) with the children (both genders) and the women ate after. Not that there was this law that women would eat later, or that men didn't serve the food as the women ate (we are Kobras, Konkanastha Brahmins, so our men help in the kitchen, but discrimination, though the least amongst communities, exists — very much), but the women were always second. So these thoughts like, 'I am a woman so I am not really good and I should always keep trying or appeasing or falling in line', may not exist in our immediate family, but it does exist around us.

As we grow up, we become super-sensitive to all the stimuli around us (especially around puberty). We start inculcating feelings of inequality or inadequacy, and before we know it, it becomes an integral part of our being. We *believe* that we are undeserving — undeserving of equality, yes, but also undeserving of praise and appreciation. And the fact that some of us are lucky enough to not experience this inequality directly while growing up does not mean that we will always be guarded against this inferiority complex or feeling of inadequacy.

So we should just work at it. Know that we come from a country where women burn in the kitchen, get beaten with sticks, are paraded naked and of course killed after the sonography says ladki! Women like us, who have had equal opportunities and support from home and hearth, should never let our guard down. The biggest demon is sitting within us and it comes from sanskara, conditioning or past experiences that we may have buried so deeply inside, we are unaware of them. We play the role of criticising ourselves and put ourselves in what is supposedly our place by mirroring the perception of inadequacy in society. Not being able to accept compliments is just one consequence.

If you are a woman who feels that her friends/partner/ parents/children don't compliment her, then you need to do some soul-searching. Have you been so preoccupied with what you think are your faults/limitations, that you haven't really noticed the compliments? Or have they actually been saying nice things to which you've not really been receptive? And lastly, when compliments do come your way, do you accept them with a kind 'Thanks' or act needy and say things like, 'What, no! I've only lost five kilos'; or 'Really? I haven't even lost two hundred grams on the scale'.

We need to finally reach a point where we are kind enough to appreciate our own efforts. Efforts need appreciation and not reminders that, uff, Dilli abhi dur hai!

The 'I don't want anyone to know that I'm on a diet' phenomenon

For the first time in my life I was having the thrill similar to that of having an illicit affair. Here I was at a posh Delhi ladies' (high-society types) lunch, going around as the 'high priestess of good food and size zero' (please don't ask me what that means, that's how I was introduced before the talk). Earlier that day, two of my clients who belong to this close-knit 'difficult to get into circle', had BBm'd me — 'Pls act as if you don't know me, if the chairperson introduces you to me'. Gosh! Why? I would've thought they'd want to flaunt their personal connection with 'the high priestess'. The reply: 'Are you crazy? I don't want anybody to know that I am on a diet!'

There, my bubble as India's 'most sought-after dietician' burst. Not one but *both* my clients wanted me to act as if I didn't know them — even though one of them was actually instrumental in getting the group to invite me for the talk! The 'I don't want anybody to know that I am on a diet' phenomenon is not uncommon. There are many reasons, ranging from the fact that diets and workouts are popular party gossip, to the fact (sadly) that we are almost ashamed or guilty that we are actually spending money on ourselves. I mean, if we spend on the latest Hermes bag or chunky diamond ring, we can fool ourselves into believing that it's a 'family heirloom', or the least we should do for 'family status'. But what about eating right? You don't owe that to family status or the next generation, so how dare you?

The 'ideal woman' thinks only about family, children, husband (not necessarily in this order) and their food, health, well-being, etc. It's only the REAL woman who knows that to keep home and hearth in order, she needs to be in fab shape and have the fitness (mental and physical) to not get unnecessarily bogged down by daily (ever-increasing) needs of the kids and family. Of course to stay in great shape she will need to eat right and get professional help if required. So make your choice, you want to be real or ideal?

Running after 'results'
Real life example

I was getting an unsolicited motivational talk from a client, Deepika, who heads HR at an equity fund. 'Listen, this is my last hope. I have no face to show. I have wasted toooo much money on all this (weight loss fads and diet). Now you HAVE to give me results. You're the only one who can do that. If I don't see results, I just lose motivation. You can do it, Rujuta. You can give me results.'

'Wait a minute. What results?' I asked.

'What do you mean?' she shot back impatiently. 'Weight loss! And quick. I don't have much time. As it is, waiting to get an appointment with you wasted so much time. Now at least the results should be quick. I am sure you can do it. You charge a bomb, babe!'

This was not the first time I was hearing this. Nevertheless, I subjected her to my well-rehearsed answer: Just like happiness, good health cannot be bought.

'Can you elaborate on that?' Deepika cut me short. My team had nicknamed her 'can you elaborate on that'. She had consistently repeated the phrase while we explained to her (in detail) the appointment procedure, waiting time, what to expect while on a package, how she could take these two months forward…. Would you like a glass of water? Can you elaborate on that?

So I did elaborate. 'Good health is priceless, it cannot be bought. You need to work at it constantly. It needs effort. Your effort. Enough effort to eventually make it effortless. You are paying me to educate you about good eating habits and to work with you to find ways to eat right given your hectic schedule. Which means that you're not paying me two rupees (or any other denomination) per gram of weight lost.'

'So? Does that mean that I have wasted my money?'

'Can you elaborate on that?' (Wow!! I had managed to win the competition in my office. I had actually asked 'Can you elaborate on that', 'Can you elaborate on that?')

'I need results! Weight loss.'

'I'm sorry, then yes, you *are* wasting your money. Weight loss should come free. You shouldn't need to pay anything for it.'

'Elaborate on that?'

'Okay, diarrhoea and dysentery can result in weight loss. You don't have to pay to get diseases. The latest and most exotic one is swine flu. Swine flu can give good results. Results = weight loss. I can't. What I will essentially do is help you gain weight.'

'WHAT??'

'Sit down Deepika, and let me elaborate. Have you seen the movie *Kuch Kuch Hota Hai*?'

'Yes. But what does it have to do with anything?'

'You know what you need in your body so that kuch kuch happens? Metabolically active muscle tissue. Muscle occupies very little volume in your body compared to fat and has the property to contract and send electrical impulses. You can grow denser muscle and a better network of nerves around it if you work out regularly, eat right, sleep right and think right. The diet plan that we come up with together will pretty much encourage you to avoid diet or food accidents, take to regular exercise and have a regular sleep/waking-up pattern — all of which will make you gain weight. Denser muscles and denser bones = weight gain.'

'Okay, I am kind of getting a grip on this. Tell me more.'

'Cool, so we are on the same page now (I love dishing out corp lingo to corp types). Deepika, a gain in lean body weight — that's the weight of your bones and muscles — is like reversing the process of ageing. As age progresses and inactivity sets in, our muscles shrink and our bones get hollow or brittle, so you lose lean body weight (LBW) and that all-important ability to keep your fat stores burning. End result? Total gain in body weight as a result of weight loss.

'Now if you equate results with weight loss, then it just makes things difficult for you. You will put an effort into eating right, working out, regularising bedtime and stuff so you will look better, feel better, your body volume will shrink, everybody around you will start telling you that you have lost weight and you will end up feeling stronger and more energetic than ever before. But then if these changes don't come with a shift in the weighing scales you feel like a loser, because you still don't have the "results" you signed up for.'

'So now what?'

'Now we just work at what is within our reach and forget about "results". Especially about putting a deadline for results. Once your body receives the right nutrients at the right time, it will start prioritising the repair work that it wants to bring about in your system. It's best that you leave this to inner wisdom and not interfere with this process. So if your body wants to take care of depleted nutrient stores, optimise hormonal response, grow denser bones, teeth, nails or hair, you let it be. You should feel confident that your body will never work against you. It will continue to drop fat stores through this process, but just because this is not reflecting on the scales it doesn't mean that it's not happening. See, we are often unaware of the fact that we are breathing or that the earth is moving around the sun, but just because we are not conscious of the process, it doesn't mean that it's not happening. It's still happening. You are breathing, right?'

'Ya, I just never thought of it this way. But it makes sense. So my money is safe. Thank you.'

The elaboration had ended, but I added, 'So the "take-away" here is that weight loss is not proof of fat loss or better health.'

'But how do I evaluate my progress? Will it ever, finally, eventually lead to weight loss or are people like me doomed to stay fat?'

'Well, as long as you *feel* light, know that you are getting lighter on the fat stores. See Deepika, learning to eat right is about dropping tension that you carry in your mind and body, and not about dropping weight. **So if you feel lighter in body and mind, you no longer need the weighing scale to validate the fact that you are on track.** But do yourself a favour and don't take it up like a project that you need to deliver within a timeline. Be as compassionate with your body as it has been with you. Heard this song? The one Kamal Haasan sings from the roof of a bus — *Jitne bhi tu karle sitam, has has ke sahenge hum, yeh pyaar na hoga kum, sanam teri kasam....* So motivation to treat the body well should be unconditional.

The love your body has shown you is unconditional no matter what you put her through — starvation, late-night binges, fad diets, all of it ya. She stood by you through everything. Payback time now.'

The gym punishment

There's a girl in the gym I go to who walks in at 6 a.m. (the gym opens at 5.30) and leaves at 9.45 — that's 9.45 at night. And that too when she's practically pushed out by the trainers because the gym closes at 10 p.m. Maybe it's partly to do with her being an aspiring actor and wanting to network in the gym, but a lot of us struggling with weight loss do tend to stay in the gym for two, two-and-a-half hours at a stretch. The truth is, anything more than a sixty-minute workout will lead to a loss of muscle tissue; this leads to a lower metabolic rate, which means that you're burning less fat through the day. Basically, exercising for more than an hour actually defeats the purpose of exercise — the exact opposite of what you're aiming for takes place. It's not a maths equation where, if you lose y amount of calories in an hour, you'll lose y x 2 calories if you work out for two hours. There's a lot of chemistry, biology and biomechanics involved. Consider what part of your body is taking the strain of over-exercise, what fuel you're burning, fat or muscle. Is it actually helping your blood circulation or making your body weaker?

Exercising is a way of loving your body, not punishing it. And spending more than an hour in the gym is like two-timing someone you love. Cheating on someone is never easy on the mind, body or senses, so it's no surprise that if you over-exercise, your body will show it — and not in the way you want. The point of exercise is that you should look like you've worked out, like you're toned, whether you're in your work clothes, saree or a salwar kameez. Instead, you'll have the kind of body where people will ask you if you've been ill.

Slave to the weighing scales

'Don't look at me like that,' said Praveen.

'No, I'm not looking at you. (Actually, I was glaring.) Do you really think I'm ever going to ask you mera wajan kyon nahi kam ho raha hai?'

He smiled sheepishly and nodded. I had signed up for personal training with Praveen and he was putting me through the rigmarole of checking my body weight. Why was I giving him a dirty look? Because on three different weighing scales in the gym, my weight had gone from 52.5 to 51 and finally 50 kilos. 'Yippee, I have lost weight!' should have been my delighted response.

Instead I was going into a zone of 'why do women practically put their life on hold for this dumb thing' and other 'how we make a mountain out of a molehill' issues. The problem was, I couldn't afford to do that. I was running late and had a workout to finish.

There are two *big* problems with checking body weight: 1) The weighing scales are *never* accurate. 2) And this is the bigger one — body weight is in *no* way an indicator of your health, fitness or beauty. I think we pretty much understand the first problem. My clients often inform me how they weigh X on their bathroom scales, Y on their gym scales and Z on their doctor's scales. To add a little more fun to their lives, they want to check their weight on my scales. When I say I don't have one, they demand to know what kind of a dietician's office is this if it doesn't even have a weighing scale. Instead of answering them, I ask if they'd like some jasmine chai. 'Jasmine tea, by the way, is a great relaxant. A relaxed state of mind is imperative for the success of the meal plan that I will suggest post the chai.' My standard line.

When you are relaxed, you generally don't behave harshly with yourself. I mean, as women, we have been brainwashed into always being nice to others, especially after marriage, but we're never told not to behave 'rudely' to ourselves. So we are all guilty of doing tons of emotional atyachar on ourselves daily. But when we feel relaxed we are willing to go easy on ourselves. So no weighing scales but jasmine chai. Tumhare paas kya hai? Mere paas jasmine chai hai!

Okay, jokes apart, families have been broken, money has been laundered, health has been lost and the body has been put through near-death experiences — all to see some elusive number on a weighing scale. One of my clients lost her mother due to a complication post liposuction (she wanted to lose weight quickly for her son's wedding). Her story almost killed me. I mean, what's wrong with us? Whom are we trying to please, and at what cost? I couldn't have possibly lost 2.5 kilos in less than thirty seconds — that's about the time I took to hop from one scale to another. And yet I know that it's standard practice in the gym for women to get themselves checked on all three weighing scales so they have yet another thing to whine about. Oh! Only three hundred grams? What, still sixty-seven?

Let's look at it this way — just because you have never had a showdown with your mother-in-law, is it safe to assume that you love her? No? There you go. The number on the weighing scale is as much an indicator of health, fitness and beauty as the absence of a showdown is an indicator of love. Or standing first in class an indicator of smartness. Even schools are now adopting more holistic and inclusive methods to assess the progress of children — shouldn't our fitness/weight-loss plans do the same? What are these holistic ways? Actually, you will just *know* whether you are doing well or not; you won't need a scale to tell you. I bet you're thinking that this whole 'you-will-just-know' thing is too out there. Okay, let's try and put it in words:

1. Are you waking up fresher?
2. Have your cravings decreased?
3. Are you feeling lighter in your body?
4. Are you feeling inspired to exercise?
5. Are your nails growing faster than the scheduled manicure appointment?
6. Is your skin feeling and looking fresher? Have the blemishes and acne decreased?
7. Do you feel like catching up with friends/family more often?
8. Do you feel like shopping (for clothes for yourself)?
9. Are you feeling hungry often?
10. Are you smiling often?

If you answered in affirmative to most questions, congrats, you are in love with yourself. Tougher than being in love with your partner/parents/children/pet, etc. And you are also on the way to losing fat the right way. The right way being the one that is doable, sustainable and enjoyable. You have set yourself free from moronic activities like checking your body weight and are ready to enjoy life to its fullest.

So now what should we do with our weighing scales? THROW them away. And if your raddi wala is willing to buy it, sell it, add Rs 1000 to that amount from my behalf and donate the money to a good cause. It will make you feel lighter. Weighing scales belong to a bygone era, not to the woman of today. So don't let your happiness or sadness depend on a number, move on. There's more to life.

Now what's the jasmine chai connection? If you've answered 'yes' to most of the questions above, you are actually experiencing a fairly good degree of calmness. A calm mind mobilises fatty acids and uses body fat as the most preferred fuel (to sustain metabolism). This way it spares the lean body tissues, keeping you not just 'light' on stress but also on the scales. Now you know why I choose the chai and not the scales.

'I need something drastic right now!'

'Eat all the time? Eat according to the four principles? You must be kidding! Look at my size. I am ninety-eight kilos and just two years ago I was more than a hundred. You have no idea what all I have done to lose weight: enema, starvation, lime shots, dudhi juice, needles poked in my body, puked dinner after eating it, worked out till I fainted, didn't eat till I fainted and now you want me to *eat*?'

'Why don't you want to? You prefer fainting or throwing up food to sensible eating?' I asked.

'No, it's not that. I am prepared to die to eat normally, but I think before that I must knock off at least twenty-thirty kilos. Once I knock that off, trust me I will eat whatever you ask me to and as many times as you want.'

'Great, then what are we doing right now? If you feel that you must be doing "drastic" things to knock off "initial weight", this is the wrong place.'

'Don't say that. I have tried everything.'

'That's exactly my point Aliya, you have tried everything and most of it — in fact all of it — was drastic. You have fluctuated, gaining all the weight you lost, and worse, yo-yoed that way several times. Seriously, I think the most "DRASTIC" thing that you can do now is EAT. And eat as normally as you would if you were ten/twenty/fifty kilos lighter.'

What I hope I made Aliya understand is that loving your body, totally and unconditionally accepting it, and being willing to nourish it with good food is the only way to lose fat and improve muscle tone, or as it's popularly called, 'lose weight'. These drastic measures that we adopt to lose the 'initial weight' only lead to drastic damages to the body, the worst being a perpetually shifting body weight. And, much like the Indo-Pak peace talks, where you take one step forward and two steps backward, you always land up in a situation worse than where you started off.

Obsessing over old jeans
'Throw them out.'

Parul looked startled. 'Come on, Rujuta. Kuch toh marker hona chahiye. Don't stand on the weighing scale, don't go by the weighing scale, so what do I go by? I should have my old jeans for that no?' It was our first meeting and Parul had gone gaga about *Don't Lose Your Mind, Lose Your Weight* for the first fifteen minutes, but then came down to business. She wanted to lose weight and had thoroughly understood that she shouldn't 'hold herself to ransom' with the weighing scales.

'So are you looking at an alternative place to hold yourself to ransom?'

'Am I really? That sounds terrible.'

'Ya, but I think that's exactly what you are doing.'

'No, Vaishali said she did the two-month programme with you and doesn't know how much weight she lost, but she now fits into jeans she wore in college. And that's why I joined. I have kept my jeans from high school too, right in the front of my wardrobe to motivate myself. I

HAVE to fit into them. It's size twenty-eight, I am now wearing thirty-six (sad face).'

'So for how long have you tangoed them in front of your wardrobe for motivation?'

'I got them in '95, so I've had them forever now, but honestly, it's only after Vaishali showed off that she can fit into her college jeans that I brought mine out.'

'And have you lost weight in these six-seven months?'

'No, but I booked an appointment with you, so that's a good start.'

'Okay, so now throw them out.'

'Why?'

'Because I want to make things easy for you (and for myself). Look, staring at jeans that are now almost from the Stone Age makes us feel ancient and that really doesn't help. Our body changes, it's inevitable, you've got to make peace with it. All you need to figure out is how much (and how many) of those changes are natural and how much of it is just circumstantial.'

'Circumstantial bole ga toh?'

'Bole ga toh, enforced. Matlab, see, what were you eating in '95? What were your activities in '95? What were your stresses in '95? Where were you staying in '95? What were your responsibilities in '95? How much time did you have for yourself in '95? Were you exercising in '95? Was it your responsibility to ensure that everybody in the household is eating and on time?'

'Yes, the circumstances under which I had a waist of twenty-eight were SOO different.'

'There you go. So don't put those jeans there; simply figure out how much of '95 you can recreate, that will bring you closer to that slim-fit, narrow waist twenty-eight jeans. Can you spare at least half the time to exercise? At least eat half as often? Can you cut back on your current stresses, at least a bit? Can you be a little more responsible towards yourself — at least half the sense of responsibility that you have towards your kids, husband, in-laws, keeping a clean kitchen, wardrobe, etc.?'

'Come on ya! It's not just that!! Okay, I mean I have been kind of a kitchen goddess and all that. So okay I own up to it. But let's be real. I was twenty-four in '95. I am touching forty now. Age is a factor too. Let's blame age. No?'

'No. Let's thank age. It teaches us — if we are willing to learn — that hanging on to old jeans doesn't help, giving up on them does. Age only means body changes, it doesn't mean it deteriorates. Whether it changes for the better or for worse is up to you. Kareena looks younger and sexier today than she did five years ago.'

'Ya, she is gorgeous. But please, she is just about thirty!'

'Okay, how about Saif?'

'Okay ya, he definitely looks hotter by the day. And now that you say it, even Shah Rukh tweeted that he can do more with his body now than he did fifteen years ago.'

'See, there you go! I say that about my body too. My mind, my body, both are calmer, stronger, better than they were fifteen years ago.'

'Ya, you're thirty-something too.'

'Yes, but I am talking of fifteen years irrespective of age; and I see that with all my clients no matter what their age. Should I tell you the secret? Ready for this?'

Deep breath, eyes closed, 'Yes.'

'Here goes: treat your body like it's not yours, treat it like it's somebody else's and you have it on rent for a while. Puzzled? Think about it as something really expensive that a friend has lent you and you can use it to get all you want and desire. You only have to look after it in return. It's like, if I give you my car, you would drive it at least ten times more carefully than how you drive your car. Drive it slower over speed-breakers, return it with a full petrol tank, have the right amount of air in the tyres, not jump signals etc.?'

'Ya...'

'With our own car, the minute we think "this is mine", that sense of ownership — instead of making us more responsible — makes us irresponsible. We will do things that we know are clearly wrong, that we would never do with someone else's. So get out of the age-old "age excuse". **Use your body like a "single hand-driven Parsi-owned car".** Get more responsible towards it, at least with things that you clearly know are wrong. Those things that you would not do with someone else's body — starving it/over-exercising it/making a couch potato out of it/stressing it with non-issues/kicking it with caffeine/clogging it with trans fat and processed food. Staying irresponsible with food and exercise and refusing to give up on old jeans is like full-on torture, ya.

'Also, the fact is, as you progress in the journey of getting leaner, fitter and more responsible towards your body, you don't just drop to a twenty-eight size. You get there centimetre by centimetre, dropping from thirty-six to thirty-four to thirty-two and further down. And you should celebrate the process, the journey, not the "arrival". The worst thing you can do as you progress from thirty-six to thirty-two is feel bad because you are not twenty-eight yet. Sensible and responsible is the name of the game, babe. As you move down sizes, you should jump in joy and punch your fist in the air. Better than yesterday and will be even better tomorrow. Just treat it like somebody else's body, and then buy new jeans for it after you have forsaken the sense of ownership over it.'

Never prioritising yourself

Real life example

This is one thing that knocks me out every single time. Hina was sitting across from me and showing me a picture on her BB. What do you think? she asked. What is it? was my answer. 'Oh! Jeans, che. My sis-in-law is in Antwerp and there is a thirty-five per cent sale so she clicks a picture of things she thinks I might want and if I like it she will buy it. It goes in our family business overheads.'

'But why? You can buy the same brand right in the shop below my office.'

'Ya, but it's not on sale. We Palampuri wives are trained to save our husband's money.'

'God! Now I know how you make your millions, all this chindi chori.'

'Stop joking. You can spend as you like because you earn so much.'

'Sure Hinaben, your monthly pocket money must be bigger than my annual earnings before paying income tax.'

'No no, all of us sisters-in-law have a budget approved by the family (read father-in-law, bro-in-law gang, max to max the mother-in-law or the sister-in-law who is either married to the eldest brother or just dominating), only unlimited expense on food is allowed.'

'Cool. So then why won't you make a dal for yourself every night as per the plan? You do like dal, right?'

'I do. But see, for lunch we don't make dal as all the men take a dabba, so we (assorted wives — includes mother-in-law and all co-sisters who live together) send dry lunch and nashta: thepla-shaak, khakra-moong, roti-sabzi, etc. So we don't make dal for lunch.'

'But you all eat at home, na?'

'Haan, but where to make new stuff again? We eat whatever we send in the dabba (the latest farmaish by the men folk) and then in the night we make "variety" (God! Not again). Kabhi bhelpuri then idli-sambhar or pav bhaji (this is usually dictated by the children and thankfully no gender discrimination here).'

'So, when do you eat what *you* want?'

'Never. Okay, no actually all of us eat what we want around that 5-6 p.m. time — bhajjiya, sev puri, samosa, all junk. So we all wear small size ka T-shirt and XXL ka pants, the famous Gujju saddlebags and hips. Actually I hardly eat but just look at my hips, standing up, see this? Jiggly wiggly. And if you see me without clothes, my thighs have bada bada khadda, wrong place pe dimples I have.'

'And phir bhi you will not eat the nutrients that your body needs. In fact you have all these issues because you haven't eaten what your body likes eating for the longest time.'

'I don't know what happens. We are all so skinny before marriage, then within two years we are like balloons or on our way there. Sabka side se fat starts bulging out.'

'Okay, stop talking like this about your body, you have tortured it enough with such irregularities in food, now be kind enough to stop the verbal abuse and come to the point. Why won't you eat dal at night?'

'See we make sabzi in the morning, so I can have that and I can make one extra chapatti in the afternoon, but dal I will need to make especially for myself at night. Nobody eats dal and roti-sabzi, we make variety, no?'

'Oh come on, you will make such elaborate dinners for variety's sake, and you can't make dal? It takes less than fifteen minutes! Just pressure cook it, almost zero effort.'

'But how to make only for myself?'

'Why not? Also make fresh sabzi and roti please. You and your nutritional requirements can't be less important than your kids' and family's variety entertainment dinner needs. God! Please don't tell me it's because dal is getting costlier by the day.'

'No no, we can spend on kitchen expenses.'

'Good. So go and make your dal, sabzi, roti fresh and use a small utensil. That way you will save your fuel and LPG cost. Okay? Also, understand the reason why you've got dimples (cellulite) in the wrong places. You didn't just get fat over the last few years because of excessive calories or limited exercise. It's about fuel efficiency. You've consumed too many calories and received very little nutrients in return, forcing such a deprived state in your body that the body fat is also turning toxic, and instead of evenly spreading out under your skin, it has developed stretch marks, cellulite and khaddas. It's like using a ten-person ka capacity wala kadai and making only one person's sabzi in it. Waste hua na? So much time and fuel to heat the kadai aur mila kya? Sabzi (and that too overcooked) only for one person. Getting it?'

'Kind of.'

'So that's why I'm telling you to eat a wholesome meal — roti, sabzi, dal — by 6-6.30 p.m., when all you eat is junk. Every calorie you eat will be worth the nutrients.'

'This variety is all junk or what? Even if I make it at home?'

'You really need me to answer that? Yes, Hinaben, make it more than once, max twice a week, and it's junk. Too little nutrients too many calories. One person's sabzi in a ten-people ka kadai.'

'Okay, can I eat moong dhokli? I'll eat it with sabzi separate. It's like dal dhokli. So the roti I will mix in moong ka dal. My mother-in-law loves it and so does my son. So at least then I am not guilty of making something only for myself like one maharani.'

'H –I –N – A BENNNN!'

'Slowly, slowly; I promise I will start making things for myself also, but this eighteen years ka aadat and bringing up I can't wipe away in just one meeting, na?'

I had to give in. 'Yes, okay, moong dhokli is a good start.'

'Good, and then every time I come you brainwash me slowly, and by two-three months I will make a meal for myself, guilt-free!'

As she walked out I couldn't help thinking how we have been conditioned to believe that we can buy jeans and cosmetics because we are 'worth it'. And when it comes to eating, something so basic, crucial and important to our health, we are simply not worth our own time.

Compromising on sleep

Sound sleep is the most essential, integral, non-negotiable aspect of losing body fat. I can't overemphasise the importance of a restful, peaceful sleep. It's the one thing that you must have if you want a narrower waist, flatter stomach and toned body.

Real life example

It was just over 7 p.m. and Nandini was looking washed-out and dead tired. It was our first meeting. She had woken up at 8 a.m., eaten nothing, drunk a cup of coffee and gone to the gym. Had 'grabbed a toast and egg-whites' for breakfast and drunk two-three cups of tea and one black coffee during back-to-back meetings till afternoon. Then she'd had a meeting with her chef, tasting and testing some yummy dishes he had made, thus overeating because the dishes were too delicious and anyway, 'I was so hungry by that time'. Then she had rushed through traffic, screamed at her driver, instructed the cook at home about what to make for dinner for saab, ordered the maid to make sandwiches for the kids and wash laundry that had been hanging in the bathroom for three days, also called the AC guy to get the vents cleaned. Then, as her driver parked the car, she'd rushed up to my office and profusely apologised for being fifteen minutes late. I tried to say, 'Chalta hai', but I don't think she heard. She was yawning and collapsing on my sofa. She wasn't dying or going into a coma, she was just dead tired and very sleepy.

A lot of 'career women' (a term I can't fully understand) have days that are just as hectic (sorry, normal) as Nandini's. Unis-bees ka farak. (Some of us are becoming the men we wanted to marry – Gloria Steinem.) So I had the task of telling her important things when I thought she was listening, which I was about to realise was never. She was either yawning or talking or saying, 'Sorry, I have to take this', before answering her phone.

How do I know her recall for the day? Because she had emailed it to me from her phone, in the car, while on her way to my office. The day before her appointment, I had been informed that, despite numerous calls, sms-es and emails, we were yet to receive the recall of her diet for the last three days. As a policy, we cancel appointments if we haven't received a client's recall, so I'd got hers last minute, as 'damage control', but only after we had given her office and her a lot of grief.

As Nandini sat on my sofa, yawning, I felt at a loss for words and was kind of overwhelmed by all the activity around me. Instinctively I wanted to put a blanket on her tired body, a pillow under the overworked head and let her nap for a while. But of course that was 'not done'. As I tried to say something, the phone rang again. It was her daughter on the line (she had a policy: if it's a call from her son or daughter, take it, no matter what, where, etc.), complaining that the chutney was too teekha and that Swati (the maid) had once again put Simla mirch in the sandwich. 'Okay baby, I'll get it sorted out. Give the phone to Swati,' she said while signalling 'two minutes' with her fingers to me. 'Swati, kitne baar bolna padega? Baby ko Simla mirch nahi, that's only for Baba. Aur chutney kyon teekha hua hai? Abhi usme thoda nimbu dalo aur please thoda dhyan rakho.'

Whoa!! 'Can we put the phone on silent?' I suggested when it rang again.

'Just this one call … Ya love, it's the eighteenth,' she said to her husband, and then, to me, 'Okay, I will put it on silent now.'

I was already feeling sapped of energy, and I had only spent a little over ten minutes with Nandini. 'Wow! I think you're going to go home and CRASH!' I said.

She smirked. 'That would be a sweet dream for me RD, if I could hit the pillow and sleep.'

'Why? You look like you're ready to sleep right now.'

'Ya, I am feeling sleepy and dead tired right now. In fact, that's how I feel through the day, but sleep for me is nothing less than a nightmare!'

'Why?'

'See I go back home and then there are hajjar things to do and I want to spend some good, quality time with my kids. And then by about 9.30 my kids go to bed and I go to my bedroom to finally get some "me time" and also to spend some time with my husband. I think we spend less than three hours with each other from Monday to Friday. So till about 10.30-11 I watch TV or I'm on my laptop checking emails and stuff. After that I try hard to go to bed, to sleep, sleep, sleep, but I lie down for hours, WIDE awake. I think about duniya bhar ka kaam, when all I want to do is SLEEP. It's such a struggle, I can't tell you. I feel like I'm cursed; you will have everything in life — money, husband, kids, career everything — but, hey, you won't be able to sleep. Finally, at around 3.30-

4 a.m., after having raided the fridge, and gone to the bathroom at least five times, I doze off for a bit. Then, of course, I have to wake up by 7 to get the kids ready for school, Viren comes back from squash and I have to go to the gym to work my fat ass off and then to work. It's a battleground man, full throttle. Always sleepy, and never able to actually sleep.'

'For how long have you had this problem with sleep? When was the last time you slept well and woke up fresh?'

'I can't remember. Must be long, long ago. I think I have had this issue now for more than thirteen years!'

'What?'

'Yeah, babe. Okay, are you telling me what to eat? I have to rush back.'

'You don't need a diet babe, you need a BREAK!'

'Are you kidding me? I can't afford to take one.'

'*You're* kidding me. I think what you can't afford is to go without sleep like this. And it's only going to get you fat.'

'You know I slog my ass off at the gym. I want to slap all the skinny bitches I see there. So much of working out and you saw my recall? I hardly eat. (I wanted to interject with, Ya, this recall won't do and stuff, but there was no chance.) So if I am not losing weight with no food and phatte workouts, how am I going to lose weight by *sleeping*?'

Lack of sleep (among many other things) screws up your recovery from exercise and life. Exercise 'works' on the basic premise that you will recover from the damage caused to the body while working out. If there's no recovery, fat burning comes to a grinding halt, exposing you to injuries, hormonal imbalances (hypothyroid, insulin resistance), digestion issues, mood swings and even panic attacks.

Now, just like love, money can't buy sleep either. So to sleep you really need to loosen up and take a chill pill. (I didn't use the words 'chill pill' with her. I know from experience that most moms hate that term. Especially if you say the word 'mom' immediately before or after 'chill pill'.) Essentially you need to review your priority list. Put yourself (and sleep and REST) at the top of your priority list. Yes, yes, yes we need to take it easy. It's anyway too difficult to achieve anything superlative when you are dog tired, and even if you do (luck by chance), it's almost impossible to derive any joy out of it.

So if your senses are being pulled in several different directions — bai, bachche, kaam, dhaam and the likes — they don't get a chance to get centred or to withdraw from these assumed responsibilities. (By assuming responsibility I mean Nandini's daughter could easily have removed the Simla mirch from the sandwich herself or told the maid to; the husband could have checked whether it's the eighteenth or twentieth or whatever, etc.) When the senses can't withdraw themselves from external stimuli, rest or sleep is hard to come by. Deep or peaceful sleep is when you experience 'nothing', and for this you should be blessed with the ability to withdraw.

Now for women who are pulled in all directions all day, winding down in front of the TV while lying on the bed is a strict NO-NO. You can do without knowing what Anandi, Ecchha, Carrie Bradshaw or Sagarika Ghose are upto. Worse still, you get to watch your partner while he surfs channels on the TV, doing nothing and saying nothing. Seriously, if you want to rest, switch off and sleep.

Switch off the TV, lights, BB, Mac; light a nice non-toxic, calming agarbatti/scented candle or oil; wash your feet in warm water; apply a drop of ghee/til oil to the soles of your feet; and then lie on your bed, pull a soothing chaddar over yourself and experience 'nothing'. You will wake up ready to experience everything.

And you still want to watch TV? Cool, just move it to another room. Watch it, and when you've had enough, switch it off. The slimmer the TV and the closer it is to your bed, the bigger your waist and the further your navel is from your spine. More on Nandini's story and the damage that the lack of sleep can cause to your hormones and metabolism later (Chapter 7). For now, just move the TV out.

Forgive, forget, forward

So you've just started on a diet, got stuck somewhere and can't eat Meal 4. You decide, chalo, today's diet is anyway gone, let me skip Meal 5 as well and have Diet Pepsi and pizza for Meal 6. Or you got up late on Wednesday and you had a conference call on Thursday morning, so you couldn't work out on both days, and you think, I might as well not do Friday since this week's workout plan has been bad anyway. The thing to do in both these cases, is not get disheartened. If you skipped Meal 4, it's okay, it happens. Eat your Meal 5 and 6 as if you've had Meal 4. You need to forgive yourself for these occasional slips. If you know you have a con call in the morning, go work out in the evening, or go to sleep the previous day knowing you will miss your workout. Don't feel guilty.

Look at the way we learnt to walk. We fell numerous times in the process, but did we feel bad, judge ourselves, and just continue to crawl for the rest of our lives? No, we continued to consistently work at it. Of course, one thing we can't overlook is that our support group at that point was strong: our parents and the people around us constantly encouraged us through the process. But, most importantly, we didn't judge ourselves. The same with your diet and workout plan. Falling now and then is part of the natural learning curve — an essential part in fact — and it's not unnatural. But you have to keep moving ahead and continue to follow it. Forgive and forget won't work — you have to forgive, forget and move forward.

2

A Fearless (Teen) Age

What's in the looks?

'So, how many of you hated the way you looked when you were two years old?' No hands went up. 'Three?' None again. 'Okay, six?' One hand went up. 'Really?' I asked. The girl looked down and started wriggling her toes. I had to go on, there were some four hundred girls in the auditorium. 'At eight?' Two-three hands went up. 'Okay ...' I tried to say teasingly, but even I was not fully convinced that (a) this was funny (b) they were ready to laugh at themselves. 'And at thirteen?' Almost a hundred hands up now. 'Fifteen-sixteen?' Wow! Looked like every girl there hated herself — most hands were up. 'And at seventeen?' Some hundred hands went down. Phew! And then a voice piped up, 'But Ma'am, we're not seventeen yet!' Roaring laughter. 'Oh!' I giggled too, but felt disturbed. Why? I asked myself. They look happy, they go to one of the best schools in the country, probably wear the best of clothes — even their uniform was so smart. Then why did they all hate the way they looked?

Our ad gurus and the wizards of marketing have made a killing by telling us that we are never thin enough, fair enough or tall enough. But that's fine, that's their dhanda. Sab ganda hai par dhanda hai yeh! And to be fair, advertising only reflects what is the acceptable (aspirational) norm in the society. But do we all aspire to be thin, fair and tall? Don't we have parents, teachers, family who could have inculcated better values in us? Or have they bought into the theory that thin/fair/tall is beautiful and that it is impossible to be beautiful enough? There is always a chance to get a shade fairer, an inch taller and a kilo slimmer. Scope for improvement! *Pleeease*! Give me a break!

The thing is, we are all born loving ourselves and our bodies. Little babies can't take their eyes off their toes, fingers, etc. And oh it's just so normal. So NORMAL to love our own body, and accept her exactly the way she is. Not lighter, fairer, slimmer. Nothing. Beautiful, gorgeous, exactly the way we are. Unconditional love. Unconditional acceptance.

Then gradually it becomes normal to be unhappy with our appearance. We start complying to set ideals of beauty! What a shame. We come from the land of Sanatan dharma, where diversity is considered beautiful. Thirty-three crore gods, each one beautiful, glorious, divine. One dark with a pink tongue and skulls around the neck, one a shy, demure virgin on the dead body of Shiva, one an old woman with a frail body, one in white on a swan or a bright pink lotus!

What happens to us from the age of thirteen onwards (for some of us, as early as seven-eight) or as we reach adolescence/pre-puberty? To me, all the Welham School girls, each one of them (no jokes), looked STUNNING! And despite this, they felt inadequate already. Why?

Teenage — the age of misinformation

Puberty is a natural but delicate phase in our lives. We

don't really grow new limbs, energy systems, hormones or anything at all during this phase. The body simply increases or decreases levels of hormones according to the gender that you belong to. So girls see a surge in estrogen and progesterone levels, and boys in their testosterone levels.

The period when you enter adolescence can pretty much determine whether you will lead your life feeling fulfilled (mostly) or feeling inadequate (mostly). This is the time when activities you take up or quit, the food you eat or refuse to eat, actually determine the course of your life. The body changes too, but that's not really an issue (it's only natural, you see). If you eat too much junk and exercise very little or not at all, this is the time you will balloon out of proportion, develop stretch marks, acne, etc. But that's hardly the point. Because whenever you want, you can change things. **The body will alter the minute you change your eating and exercise habits** (people like me make a living from this fact). What causes delays in the process or makes the journey difficult is your personality. If the body and mind have been well nurtured with regular physical activity (at least sixty minutes of hardcore exercise a day, on most days of the week), and nourished with fresh and hygienically-prepared food, then the changes that puberty brings about in the physical body are smooth and natural. The hormonal changes make the mind and body very sensitive to the environment around. So as teenagers we need to look at exercise and good food as building material for our personality and life.

The lack of good food and exercise and irregular sleep and waking times inhibit our mental, physical and spiritual growth. The heart, kidney, liver, lungs, intestines, height, muscle mass, bone density, hormones, enzymes, every single cell and function in the body don't grow/operate to their optimum capacity. Growth suffers, making you prone to illnesses and imbalances (physically and mentally) later in life.

This is the time when elders in the family need to do a lot of hand-holding so that we experience a smooth transition into adulthood. With the joint family now almost non-existent, the burden is almost entirely on our parents. Traditionally, large joint families would be packed with aunts and cousins, who were almost your age or just a bit older, to whom you had 24 x 7 access and could share all the pains, discomforts and agonies of growing up and that too without being judged. The nuclear family, with working parents, has made *car* possible and *sanskar* difficult (line borrowed from swamiji of Parmarth ashram). Having access to and the love and understanding of a trusted adult is of paramount importance at this time. Even the traditional gurukulam system, where one was sent at the age of seven, was a way to receive love, guidance and understanding of your body, mind and life itself from a guru.

Why is access to a trusted adult, love and understanding so important? It's in this phase of life that you need guidance and support, because mentally you lack the ability to decipher and digest the changes that the body goes through hormonally.

Aggression

Many teenagers feel an undue aggression that manifests in their slamming doors, shouting at their mothers, or worse, in eating disorders. If you feel angry and have a lot of hostility, don't worry, these are perfectly normal feelings. (And mothers, please don't feel guilty thinking you haven't brought your child up properly.) The anger and resentment comes from things we don't fully understand — why do girls take second place in the world, what's going on with our vagina, why am I so angry if someone touched me a certain way.... Ideally, we would have an open environment where we can talk about these things. But till we have that safe environment, just know that it's okay: don't be angry with yourself for feeling angry. You're part of an adult world the mechanisms of which you don't yet fully understand. You just need to arrange those feelings in your head and channelise them. The best strategy would be to play a sport or learn a creative art. Playing a sport channelises this anger through a competitive spirit; pursuing an art like dance allows this aggression to emerge as creative energy.

What's so special about eight?

Though puberty is natural, it's also very special and eventful, almost like a turning point in your life. Little wonder then that every religion marks this phase in our life with a special ceremony. Hinduism has the thread ceremony, Christianity has communion post the age of eight; Islam Judaism, Buddhism, Baha'i, Zoroastrian — you name it, almost every religion acknowledges that coming of age or entering puberty is a crucial time in our development (physically, mentally, spiritually) through some ritual or celebration around the age of seven-eight. Why, even atheists conduct group training or admit only children above the age of seven or eight into their life skills or ethical training camps.

Why have a ceremony or a community acknowledgement that you are now 'coming of age' or 'grown up'? It's a way of easing our journey into adulthood; it's a way of acknowledging that you are now an individual and that you should gain knowledge (all kinds, including religious) and social skills to be a part of the adult world.

The entire point of such ceremonies was to prepare us mentally to take on physical changes and challenges in our stride. It really was meant to teach us to go beyond physical limitations (including gender) and to do our dharma towards ourselves, family and community in a righteous and fearless manner. Today, we sadly have retained only the symbolic and the ritualistic part of it, while the true meaning has been lost.

And why have all this jazz around eight? Simply because we start sexually maturing around this age. Ya, ya, I know your jaw has dropped and your mother is telling you that there is no truth in this statement, but it is a valid fact. The process of course may take up to four years (sometimes longer), but the journey has begun.

The beginning of the end!

Is this marked with the end of the angelic childlike innocence? Nope. But it is marked with an increased awareness about your sexual organs and your body. The pineal gland in the brain (eyebrow centre) starts sending signals to various hormones in the body, and they start increasing or decreasing depending on your gender. Typically, this is the phase when you start hating boys (simply because they are boys, nothing personal) and little boys start using the gents' loo instead of following mama to the ladies'. You see what I am saying — awareness about your gender.

This is the time when our hormones change and confusion prevails in the mind at all times. Are you grown up or are you a little child? Sensible parenting, all-round development in school and a close-knit family that rises over petty issues are priceless at this time. No, actually the priceless thing is to have a sister (this is my unshaken belief). In my work, I have often noticed that women with sisters do better at fat loss than women without sisters. What do sisters provide? Love, support and patience, things that we don't always provide ourselves. (So your sis will be cool with you but may be damn harsh on herself.)

So now what does all this have to do with diet/food/nutrition, etc.? Well, if you see my point, everything. This is the age when you start thinking of yourself as a 'girl' instead of a 'child'. Now that you are a girl, you subconsciously pick up on conditioning prevalent in the society about what you are supposed to be like and start complying (sadly, mindlessly) with it. So you learn that you must not laugh loudly, jump from such a height, hang from a bar for fun or let your chaddi show while sitting — all this is bad manners, please. The worst thing is that these messages are so subtle that your parents, family, community, school don't even realise that they're forcing you to become part of the production line called 'good, cultured girl'. Every time I hung from the ledge in his home in Girgaum chawl, Appa, my grandfather, would say, 'Langdi jhalis tar lagna hoycha nahi.' Which simply meant that if I fell down and broke a leg, nobody would want to marry me. That was the big danger, that I would be left to kato my life unmarried; leg broken or not was not such a big deal!

Religion, schooling, family upbringing — all these should instead encourage you to be your own person, the person that comes naturally to you, and allow you to express your swabhav in a safe and organised environment. You don't have to be delicate, you don't have to be shy, you don't have to be bad at math and you don't have to be fair and you definitely don't HAVE to be thin!

See my point? You don't have to be thin or any particular size for that matter. In fact, there is a good chance that you may appear slightly plump, with a little bump on the stomach, and feel a bit awkward about your appearance. It's just that your organs are growing and hormones are surging. Soon you will have your first period (so technically you are ready to reproduce). So there we are, with the brains, tantrums and the understanding of life of a little child and the body of a well-endowed woman, almost. It's the almost part which makes us look (we think) ugly and feel (truly) awkward. Hair appears at random places, all of a sudden you get conscious about wearing your pink spaghetti Barbie top or roaming around at home in a petticoat. In a matter of three-four years, our body becomes that of a full-grown adult and our mental capacity sadly still sucks. And call it cruel, but this is exactly the time when it matters like hell that you EAT RIGHT!

Tracking weight

You know what often strikes me about growing up? Till the age of six or eight, children feel a sense of pride that their weight is going up, and measuring their height is a fun activity. My sister and I tracked our heights on an almost weekly basis, so the wall behind our bedroom door had pencil marks and dates where the top of our heads reached. (It also had the heights of all our cousins and the children of some of my mom's friends.) No matter how insignificant the height gain, we felt really happy that we were growing and that our weight was going up too, though the latter wasn't something that could be measured with as much frequency (thank god my mother was too middle-class and didn't own a weighing scale). So our weight got checked only when we were at a railway station and if there were two fifty paisa coins accessible and if the train was running a bit late and the platform was not too crowded and, most importantly, only if the machine was working! Too many variables. So our weight got checked once in six months and there was always an increase. Yippee. Then after we got our periods, we almost got critical of our growth. We cringed every time the weight went up and we were seriously unhappy that our height was not increasing as much, so unhappy that we eventually gave up on measuring our heights! Soon tracking our height and weight was no longer fun or a time pass, but a way to feel defeated/inadequate. Not thin enough and not tall enough.

Mother – the ultimate enemy

Now read this carefully. If you have nursed a food fad or fear at this age, or thought of yourself as 'too fat', then you are likely to make it tough for yourself as an adult to lose weight (i.e. reach optimum body composition or lose fat mass). Why would you think of yourself as fat? Now I hate saying this, but if you have a mother, or you are being a mother who gently nudges your daughter's (valid for son too) tummy and 'encourages' her to stay off fries/

chips/burgers/papad/rice/banana, etc., only one signal is being sent out. Fat is ugly and thin is beautiful. Thin finds acceptance and fat finds rejection. Research says that we are most sensitive to criticism that comes from our mothers, followed by sisters, and later dads, brothers, etc. Need proof? Really? Whom do we hold maximum grudges against — mom or dad? Whom do you never forgive easily — mom or dad? From whom do you 'expect' irresponsible behaviour — mom or dad? If your father or sibling called you motu/fatso/chubbu, it's okay, they are all idiots. But if your mother called you that? How could she? The bitch! *Or* — Oh no! I am adding to my mom's already troubled life by having a little tum-tum around my waist, I must be a really bad girl.

Often, girls who go on a 'diet' at this age are only expressing a need to be loved and accepted by their families. It's an expression, more often than not, of their mother's insecurities and fears. A Marathi saint once said, 'Swami tinhi jagacha aai bina bhikari', which means 'The master of all three worlds without a mother is like a beggar'. We all agree. Here's my take on this, you can't become the swami of even one world or for that matter anything at all if your mother is not mentally and physically healthy/fit. As we grow up and start thinking of ourselves as girls, we start mirroring our mother's habits and lifestyle more than ever. If she is exercising and eating right, there is a good chance that you will too. If she is busy calling you fat and being irresponsible about her eating habits, there is a good chance that you will too. If she is at peace with her menstrual cycle and has an open dialogue with you about it, you feel naturally comfortable about it and know that you can always bank on her in case of doubts. If she is awkward/shy/superstitious about it, then you too will have issues/pains/discomfort with your menstrual cycle.

'Please get her thin before March,' a mother pleaded with me. 'I have to show them that my daughter is capable of doing whatever she wants.'

'Get a life, Mom,' retorted the daughter. Aggression in words and tone only, because she had already complied with her mother's demand. Forgone a 'catch up at CCD in the evening' and made her way to my workplace. The daughter was going to subject herself to a diet and lose weight so that the mother wouldn't 'lose face' in front of her family. **This, I think, is the 'new-age honour killing'.** Why should you let 'society' judge your skills as a mother based on whether your daughter is five, ten or even thirty–forty kilos overweight?

In my list of things mothers should never say and daughters should never hear, 'Get her thin' comes first! The March deadline was for a wedding in far-flung Amritsar and for distant relatives who met every time somebody popped or married (hey no, it's not the same thing ;)). So why — for the people you rarely meet, rarely interact with — do you want to lose weight? Or worse still, want your daughter to lose weight? Shouldn't she lose weight for herself and only if she feels like it (or has the environment where she can safely express that she wants to lose weight without being told to)? So if your mother tells you to lose weight, wink and say, Okay momsy, let's do it together. I need your help and company. If your daughter tells you to mind your own business, say, Okay. Don't push it. Seriously.

Cellulite: 'Worse than my mom and more lethal than her taunts'

Okay, first of all, let's understand what cellulite means. It basically means a localised change in your body fat under the skin (subcutaneous fat) brought about by a change in the hormonal environment.

It usually starts after puberty, because the body is growing and changing so much, and it's completely normal, so don't worry about it or feel upset, or ugly. These changes are not ugly, in fact all of us carry cellulite so think of it as a 'puberty mark', much like a birth mark. Even boys will have it, so chill. It's just like if somebody gets a brain wave to come up with equipment/pill/cream/gel to get rid of your birth mark, then they first need to convince you that it's ugly/abnormal/uncool etc., right? So they would have yucky names for it just like they have for cellulite — orange peel or cottage cheese skin. Seriously, cellulite that you develop as a part of normal growing up doesn't look bad at all.

Anything that the body goes through which alters its hormonal environment will reflect itself as cellulite formation on the skin. Inactivity, gaining too much weight in a short span of time, too much stress, crash dieting, over-exercising, lack of sleep, etc. The thing is, if it's just a 'puberty mark' it is almost invisible, specially if you are involved in a sport or regular exercise and are good with eating habits (no junk or overeating). But if you get worked up about your puberty mark and subject it to crash dieting, kneading the area (usually pelvic area or thighs) with oils/creams/gels/machines etc., it will just grow in size and in other areas of your body too (because again you are changing the hormonal environment with drastic dieting or over-exercise).

So why take offence at something which is a normal part of growing up? Simply up your intake of essential fats like ghee, nuts, paneer; eat fresh fruits and vegetables; avoid colas and don't stay hungry for long hours or stay up too late. Also, work out regularly (same thing even if you get it as a 'pregnancy mark'). Yes, sweety, takes much more than the application of a cream or gel (and if you read the bottle carefully, it says in really small letters — exercise and diet for good results).

The missing link — nutrient deficiencies

So can I say this again at the cost of being repetitive — **what you eat at this age can make or break you as a person**. Both physical and mental well-being depends heavily on whether or not you are keeping your body well-nourished.

To keep the body well-nourished, we need to eat right (not small; see Chapter 7 for nutrition strategies). And to eat right we need some basic education about our food and body. Family attitudes and values regarding food are easily absorbed by the sponge-like adolescent mind, and whether or not we like it, have a much bigger influence than peer pressure and the school canteen. Education is the key here. (Sometimes I wonder how much it is the key to — the key to a world free from terrorism, poverty, gender bias and also obesity.)

During adolescence, we don't think of food as a means of getting nutrients. It's also at this age that it matters the most that we look good, because we are just dying to turn into a beautiful swan from an ugly duckling. But in spite of that, we just don't make the connection. Food to us becomes either something that we must eat or we must not eat in order to look good. Ha ha ha, I mean thin. Good = thin. Beautiful = thin. Gorgeous = thin. Sexy = thin. So there we go, we want to look as thin as possible and food is something that we make a fad or a fear out of so that we achieve it.

That these fads or fears we nurse could wreak our system from within (because of nutrient deprivation) is something that we ratta maro right from the eighth standard. Vitamin C deficiency = scurvy, Vitamin D deficiency = rickets,

Vitamin A deficiency = night blindness. But since we don't see anybody we know suffering from these diseases, it becomes just another thing that we learn in school, write in exam papers to score marks but see little or no application of it in life. (Just like the year in which the Battle of Plassey was fought, the amount of rabi crop grown in UP, reduction reactions or electron transfer, algebra equations, etc. Please feel free to add more from your experiences and email them to me. Let's make a Facebook page of 'things we learnt in school and never use'.)

What we *do* see all the time with people we know are mood swings, stretch marks, constant battles to lose weight, potbellies, love-handles, saddlebags, lethargy, tiredness, insomnia, PMS, depression, difficult pregnancies, random weight gain at menopause, hip fractures after bathroom falls, bad knees, lower back pains … the list is endless. But we just never link it to nutrient-deprivation or deficiencies. Boss, apne country mein, as long as you get good marks you are forgiven for not using your dimaag. So you are forgiven sweeties for not realising that, though your grandmom never got rickets, she broke her hip or thigh bone after falling in the bathroom, and the doctor put her on calcium tablets (only after the bone breakdown), indicating that maybe she didn't eat right as a child.

While we are all busy changing from state exam boards to CBSE/ICSE and of course IB now, what really needs to change is the way we think and use the knowledge that we receive in school. The board exams in your tenth/twelfth hardly matters; what matters is what you learnt and your ability to apply that learning.

Anorexia and bulimia

At the end of my address to a group of middle-class and middle-aged Maharashtrian women at a book reading club, one of them asked me 'if throwing up after eating was a good idea'. Taken aback, I asked her if she was joking or really wanted me to answer the question. 'Please answer,' she said earnestly, 'because Princess Diana has used this "method" to stay thin.' Wow! Till that moment I had gone about my life thinking being a middle-class, middle-aged, Maharashtrian and a member of a book club made you immune to fads and fears related to food and obsessions about the body. Just because a 'celebrity' has done it, doesn't make it the right thing to do. But that's the kind of following and effect they have on people. If my favourite superstar wears a certain chaddi-baniyan, so will I.

Alright, coming back to the point. Throwing up food after eating is a psychological disorder called bulimia, not eating anything at all (starvation) or eating very little is another disorder called anorexia. Both are conditions where the person affected is looking to gain love, approval and acceptance; it's a deeper emotional issue manifesting itself as fear of food.

The problem here is that long periods of starvation are often followed by episodes of stuffing or overeating. This makes the person feel worse and she punishes herself by putting herself through another long period of starvation, only to eat a lot again. So she goes from being a 'good girl' (starving) to a 'bad girl' (eating) all the time. In bulimia, it's not just starving and stuffing but even throwing up, depleting the body of its nutrients and the all-important vitamin B. Whether it's bulimia or anorexia, the affected person is seriously in trouble and drained out waging this constant battle against natural urges to eat and to stay thin.

Much against the popular perception, anorexic and bulimic people are largely fat and not skinny. And even if you belong to the tiny minority who is skinny, your basic health and well-being is at stake. Sadly, a lot of popular weight loss diets — even those churned out by qualified dieticians — are almost anorexic in nature. Eventually, your body forces you to give in to your natural urge to eat. Unfortunately, by this time you've probably lost the understanding of where or when to stop eating. At all times, remember that a 'diet' should comprise food and encourage you to eat, not the exact opposite.

Anorexia and bulimia, which was once confined to the super rich or teenagers, is now fast spreading amongst the middle-class, middle-aged, intellectual crowds too. Weight loss industry, take a bow! Common sense, bow out please.

All about periods

At yet another girls' school, I wrote down all the things that my audience (eighth to tenth standards) told me they associated with food. This is what it read like: *Food = Binge. Starve. Anorexia. Skinny. Fat. Thin. Chubby. Guilt.* Nothing to do with nutrition or growth. Nothing at all. Only fads and fears. But that's fine. Yeh umar hi aisi hai. All this is allowed as adolescents. What is not allowed is to leave girls (and boys) directionless. Information is the only way to provide direction sans judgment. Typically, all that we get (as girls go on a hormone rampage) at this age is, 'Don't eat this/Don't go so close to your cousin/ Don't stare at that boy like that/Don't stare at yourself in the mirror for such a long time'. Uff. Can we instead just get some real information on what to expect instead? As in why, in the first place, we have all of a sudden such an interest in our bodies, appearance; why at this age we start playing games like flames, become ardent 'fans' of some film stars, etc. They even have songs, kahavate, cocky dialogues for this age. 'Garam jawani', 'bali umar', 'sola saal ki nazuk kali' etc. In Marathi there's a song — *Solawa waarish dhokyacha* — the age of sixteen is dangerous.

This 'dangerous' interest in our bodies is because we have either started menstruating or are about to start menstruating. And the problem is that we don't know much about menstruation. All we know is that our body is changing rapidly, and most of the time we are pretty clueless about how to come to terms with it. All our 'information' comes from friends, older cousins, trashy magazine columns or other unreliable sources. I knew that I would start bleeding and then I would wear a pad, like the one I saw on TV, which absorbs blue ink. I was told I am lucky because, before the advent of pads, little girls would spend hours in the bathroom washing their special cloth or kerchief which substituted for the pad. But they couldn't throw it away; they had to wash it while their stomachs would cramp, heads would feel dizzy and backs would pain. Then they would go through the embarrassment of putting that cloth to dry, away from the prying eyes of their brothers, fathers, uncles, visiting relatives etc., and hell would break loose if it wasn't dry before they needed it. But now with the pad it's easy, use and throw, rejoiced a friend from tenth standard while I was still in the eighth.

The glee on her face was too much for me and the entire description of the first period was like *yuuuck* (my generation hadn't learnt to say fuck in school)! Too traumatic. And since I didn't have the mental ability to use words to describe my feelings, I would simply make a dirty face every time anybody spoke about it. Yet I was hungry to know more. There was so much misinformation, superstition, mystery around it that 'periods' became like a 'watch it from the edge of your seat suspense thriller'. It's very painful, I was told in a matter-of-fact tone by some of my older friends. It's to prepare a woman to bear her painful life, they said, because she will experience pain when her husband lies on top of her on the first night after their wedding and when she delivers a baby. So the monthly pain was 'practice' to improve 'tolerance' levels in women for their painful lives. The period now seemed like some weekly badminton practice and labour pain during delivery like the big inter-society tournament. Difficult, tiring and important enough to win.

The girls in my school and building belonged to well-educated families, most of them had mothers like mine who were working and hence 'independent', and yet they had all accepted that pain was an inevitable part of a girl's existence and that it would only increase as she grows up to be a woman. Before I knew it, I had bought into the idea that the main aim of a girl's life was to chup-chaap bear all the pain and then deliver a baby, jisko dekh ke all the pain disappears! And to be able to deliver a baby she must bravely (read SILENTLY) go through a lot of pain every month and bleed from the place she pees.

Now I think, what *crap*!!

Our schools need to teach us as much (if not more) about food and exercise as they do about the climate of California, the sedimentation of rocks, Pythagoras theorem, Shakespeare, etc. How fit (physically and mentally) we get as citizens (global, Indian, or local) depends much more on our attitude towards food and fitness than on everything else that they teach in school and college. Like Aamir Khan says in *3 Idiots*, there is a big difference between well-trained and well-educated. An educated tiger knows that she belongs to the woods, deserves to be free, hunts freely, loves warmly and attacks ferociously. A well-trained tiger sits on a stool when ordered to.

Periods/chums/menstruation is just as natural as respiration, circulation, digestion and all the other biological/physiological processes that you learnt about in school. Are any of them painful? Hmm, only if you are sick. Normally they are smooth and you are happily oblivious of these processes. Why then do we make such a big deal about periods? Here's my attempt to solve this mystery. For starters, respiration, circulation, digestion are processes that we are used to having since birth so they are not new and hence we don't fear them. Secondly, they also occur in boys and men and not just women. So since we get periods later in life, we fear them, like one fears the unknown. What do you do when you decide to take a trip to somewhere new? You read up, talk about the place to people who have already been there and pack your bag according to the information you have gathered from trusted sources. You are now well-equipped to deal with unknown territory. We need to use the same logic with our menstruation.

During menstruation, an average amount of blood loss is about thirty-five millilitres, and it can be completely pain-free if you enjoy good levels of fitness. Just like respiration: if you climb stairs but you enjoy good levels of fitness, your lungs don't gasp or groan for air. Also like circulation: if you enjoy good levels of fitness, your feet don't swell at the end of a day where you've stood for a long time. So let's say you climbed stairs and you are out of breath, what's the first thought that crosses your mind? Ah! I need to exercise and improve on cardio. Or is it, This is fate! I have to suffer like this every time I climb stairs. Just like my mother suffers, my aunt suffers, my sister suffers, my friend suffers and my maid suffers.

Black makes you look thin?

Sorry to burst the bubble, but advice that magazines give you, like 'wear black to look thin', 'wear a T-shirt with vertical lines', is best left in the magazines. If you're carrying more weight than you should be, any colour you wear, black, green, magenta, will not disguise it. One time you should wear black though is when you're wearing that LBD and showing off your figure. If a woman who is overweight wears black, she's just going to get bitchy comments like 'Oh, she's trying to hide those tyres'. The only thing that can make you look thin is to carry less weight — whether it's on your body, or in your mind (because you think you look fat).

Another heartbreaker — don't go by those question-answer advice columns in magazines and newspapers. Here's something I would like to share with you. A year ago, I got a call from a journalist with a magazine (a leading women's mag) congratulating me for the success of the book and offering me one of their advice columns. They have a wide readership, he said, and their readers had loved my book and wanted my opinion on what they should be eating and what exercises they should do, etc. Just as I was feeling really good about myself, my ego getting massaged, he said that all I would have to do is pay 25,000 rupees for half a page. 'What! I thought you would be paying *me*,' I blurted. Anyway, though he felt he was presenting me with this wonderful opportunity to reach out to all potential clients (even a mug shot of mine would be carried with the column, he said; and I could even just come with my own questions, and give answers to those made-up questions), I declined.

I felt so cheated that this stuff happens. Through my teenage years, all my knowledge of sex, vaginas, menstruation, contraception came from all these advice columns. To think now that they're likely to be paid for and fake! The answers are just a way to sell packages!

And yes, I do write a column for a magazine (*Outlook*) now, but I get paid for it! Not enough, but I get paid nevertheless! ☺

How is it that we so clearly know that improving cardio levels will make climbing easier, or that losing weight and strengthening leg muscles will make circulation easy and we don't use fate, gender, society, mentality, etc. as an excuse to suffer? Why do we then not know that stronger muscles, flexible joints, better cardio levels, optimum body fat levels (not the same as 'ideal body weight', an outdated concept which needs to be discarded pronto) will lead to pain-free periods? Just like pain-free climbing. So there we go, painful periods is as abnormal as gasping for breath after climbing three flight of stairs or your feet swelling because you stood for three hours today. (Oops ... even as I write this I feel I may be going horribly wrong. That perhaps we have already accepted struggling for air and swollen feet as normal. As normal as PMS trouble, craving chocolate before periods or a painful first two days of periods.)

So let's first accept that we are intelligent enough to know that good fitness levels make life easier and reduce, in fact eliminate, undue pain. How do you enjoy good levels of fitness? Eat right. Eat right. Eat right. And work out. Hardcore. No walks around the building compound/garden/to school/to the parlour/to a friend's place, or worse still, 'I take the stairs'. This is full on aunty-giri! (If you 'exercise' like an aunty, you will look like one too — right shape at the wrong place: stomach will be round, butt will be flat.) You need to be slogging your ass off, challenging your body to go beyond its limitations and the mind beyond its conditioning.

To eat right you don't have to do anything spectacular or exotic. Just normal, boring things not worth discussing with friends. The simplest thing you could do is start following the Nutrition Strategies (Chapter 7) and the four principles of eating right (see Introduction), and the stupidest thing you could do at this age is 'go on a diet'. Especially if that decision to go on a diet is driven by a motivation to 'fit in'. You may be happily oblivious to the fact that you are succumbing to regressive mentality that you 'must be like this or like that'. The drive to eat right shouldn't stem from a fear of being left out in the race to look great. Instead it should stem from a love and responsibility towards your body. Obviously love and responsibility can sometimes inconvenience you a hell of a lot and make you do uncool things like carrying a dabba from home!

Women who inspire

Here are two stories that inspire me: two women who, as teenagers, went on crash diets with a great deal of 'success' and suffered so much within months that both have now dedicated their lives to teaching and spreading awareness about the physical body and the right way to treat it: with respect and not with contempt. (One of them runs a fitness studio in Mumbai, and the other a yoga centre in Delhi.)

One of these women was gifted a stay at a weight-loss farm after her tenth standard exams. She lost some twelve kilos in a week and then gained forty kilos in less than four months when she returned home. The other employed tremendous willpower and stayed on nimbu pani for six months, and one day, while sitting for a puja, her spine collapsed, just like that.

For both, the initial euphoria of weight-loss had given way to anger, sickness, frustration with the body. But they turned the tide in their favour by learning from their experiences and by letting nothing come in the way of good health and them. No, not even weight loss. Both discovered that with eating right and working out in a scientific manner, the body weight remains under control and so does health. You don't have to lose one to achieve the other.

The thing with getting thin or losing weight is that we really need to understand what the intention behind it is. Take this from me: if the intention is anything other than improving health and fitness levels, it's not worth it, not at all. If you are going to lose out on the most precious, priceless gift of good health, then you're better off staying fat! Seriously. Every programme that you take up should guarantee that you get plenty to eat so that your growing body gets complete nourishment — all the vitamins, minerals and amino acids and all the undiscovered nutrients and the goodness of seasonal foods and the special preparations for festivals. No deprivation. No crash diets. No nonsense.

What is beautiful

Ideals of beauty keep changing so trying to change according to what is currently considered 'beautiful' is foolish. While growing up, I kept worrying that my lips were not as thin and delicate as my mother's. They were big and pouty. Through a large part of my teenage years, I tried pulling my lower lip in (especially in pictures) so that it wouldn't look 'ugly'. It was quite a painful task and I was often ashamed of what some of my well-meaning aunts described as 'smart but not beautiful' looks. Later, as I grew up and took to part-time instructing at an aerobics studio during my postgraduate sports nutrition days, clients complimented me on my 'full' lips. Just seven-eight years ago, what I'd been ashamed of had become an object of admiration! People enjoyed my classes and thought I was well-toned, so then I was no longer a 'tomboy'. Flat abs, full lips were 'in'. Just like smaller hips are now in but Asha Parekh and co had to pad up theirs to look wide. And then think of some African tribes who actually keep pressing their boobs with stones or iron because a flat chest is considered beautiful. All of us are beautiful; just like Kareena says, we have an inherent beauty. We simply need to celebrate it, not hide it, pad it or contort it.

The thing about breasts

Yes, we are conscious about our body weight, complexion (we even have creams now which come with a scale to measure your 'fairness quotient' — wah kya technology hai!), size of the waist and all that, but we are most concerned/unhappy/conscious about the size of our breasts. Most of my women clients are unhappy with their breasts, especially if they are still young. Actually no, I can safely say that ALL my women clients are, irrespective of age and size of their breasts. They are either too small or too big, they are never perfect or even okay-okay. It's almost something that they are ashamed of and is somehow harming their womanhood. So why do we make a big deal about our boobs? Ask Sush, Rakhi, Pam, you say? Well, just look at the ancient sculptures and paintings of women: nothing to hide, only some jewellery to adorn their beautiful bodies, their hips and breasts in full view, round, large and just steaming hot. Raunchy? Nope. Simply an expression of the beauty in female form, uncorrupted by 'ideal' sizes, shapes, colours, etc. In fact travel all over India and look at the caves, temples and monuments and you will find in there a catalogue, almost, of breasts. Some flattish with hardened nipples, some round and big, some cylindrical and weighing down, some long and contorted. There is really no ideal shape and each one of us is different and perfect exactly the way we are.

For one, you should know that even your two breasts will differ from each other (not too much, but they will be different, same-same but different; one may be rounder, larger, lower than the other). The breast tissue is made up of fat tissue and the glandular tissue. The breast sits on top of the pectoralis (gym name — pecs; simple name — chest muscle) on the chest wall and is attached to your chest by a connective tissue called Cooper's ligaments. These act as a natural sling or bra holding your breasts. By the way, both men and women have breasts, it's just that in women they are well-developed, thanks to the hormones released during puberty. But give our laadla an environment where estrogen is higher because of high body-fat levels and inactivity, or because he's taking supplemental testosterone, and you will have well-rounded breasts in men. Come on, go to any water park or beach in India and you will find more men flashing their saggy boobies than women, and if you are wicked enough to give them some hormones you can even have them lactate. Wanna take turns breast-feeding the baby?

The anatomy

Okay, on a less bitchy note, here's some anatomy. The breasts consist of:

1. Milk glands (lobules) that produce milk
2. Ducts (like a passage) that transport milk from milk glands to the nipple
3. Nipples (which get hard on stimulation, touch, cold and even post-exercise)
4. Areola (pink to dark-brownish colour pigment around the nipple)
5. Connective tissue that surrounds the lobules and duct
6. Fat (dhan te nan...)

In general, fat women will have bigger breasts than thinner women, but then again, this is just in general. It's absolutely possible to have thin women with bigger breasts and fat women with smaller breasts. Possibly, depending on which rumour you heard first or which magazine influenced you first, you believe that there are creams, gels, exercises, diets, etc. to increase the size and change shape. NO!! That's just playing to your fears, insecurities and feelings of inadequacies. However, there is much truth in the statement 'girls with big hearts have small breasts'. That's because a sizeable part of the breast is made of fat tissue. So girls who exercise and eat right have lower body fat levels, leading to smaller breasts and big hearts, as a response to training.

Oops, oops forgot to add — the breast tissue has hair follicles. So if you have hair spurting from around the nipple, chill. It's normal, you didn't just blow your chance to marry and settle down.

I must, I must, I must increase my bust! Revives memories almost the way the nursery rhyme 'Jack and Jill' does? It's just that you rolled your arms over each other in 'Jack and Jill' and learnt the rhyme when you were three to five years old; and with the other rhyme, you brought your palms together with a vigorous action of your shoulders and learnt it when you were around thirteen-fifteen.

So a large part of my career has gone into understanding and learning to communicate this one funda effectively — that loss of body fat will result in reduction of fat from the breast tissue as well. There is NO magical way to reduce the hips, thighs and lower ab bulge while keeping the cup size intact. The human body is pretty democratic — either sab ka badhega, ya sab ka katega. Also, there is no need to fear exercises like dumbbell presses or the plank or push-ups (if you are strong enough to do a full push-up — WOW!) — they won't decrease your bust size. I think every trainer has to battle this perception in his/her life — how do I get men to work the lower body and women to work their upper body. Anyway, well-developed pecs make your breasts look nicer and reduce the load on the upper back and neck (breasts sag you see, with gravity, especially if you are big or are a victim of a 'done everything to lose weight' fad). Train your back too — upper, middle and lower; it helps your breast and hips to look nicer. In fact, train your entire body: every muscle that exists (approximately 640) is worth exercising. Wanna slap somebody hard or lift and carry your baby with ease? Develop your pecs, girl.

THE FOUR STRATEGIES

Weight loss is about improving your health, not about winning approval from your peers, or because you want to fit into that pair of jeans. Your focus should be on getting healthy and fitter — losing weight is a by-product of these. Don't start off thinking that you want to lose weight, because then you're bound to try those crash diets and over-exercise, ruining a lot of things in your body, like hormones, tendons, etc. When you take that step to getting fitter, these should NOT be the reasons:

1. I need to lose weight to wear good clothes.
2. I have such a pretty face, now if I could only lose weight I can give Ash ji some competition (a fifteen-year-old aspiring actress from Agra once said this to me).
3. My jeans fit me from the butt and not from the waist.
4. If I am not scoring well I should at least be thin.
5. I just want to look glamorous and skinny in college.
6. My boyfriend likes me thin.
7. My father/mother is a fitness freak.
8. I am getting stretch marks on my butt/thigh.
9. I wanna show them.
10. Thin is in.

Here is a summary of the four strategies for Nutrition, Exercise, Sleep and Relationships during this age. For details, see Chapter 7.

Nutrition strategies	Exercise strategies	Sleep strategies	Relationship strategies
Learn to identify junk food so that you are not making the big mistake of consuming it every day. Don't use food as something you will eat (or not eat) to get back at your mum or to prove a point to 'others'. Canteen food is, well, canteen food. Carry food from home on most days. And if YOU do it, it becomes 'cool', right!	Learn a classical art form — dance/ music/ painting — whatever may be your calling. It works at expressing many emotions which you may not have developed the tact to verbalise in the 'adult' world. It leads to fewer 'Big deal!' and storm-out sessions with parents. Learn a sport, one which requires you to be outdoors, to develop your kinesthetic intelligence. Learn inversions like headstand, hand stand, shoulder stand to develop the strength (mentally and physically) to go against conventions or conditioning.	Late nights are cool as long as they are not an everyday affair. Just like learning to identify junk, learn to identify toxic or junk night-outs. Do the ones you like doing and self regulate the frequency — best way to look skinny. Too many late nights (whether pyjama party/ studying/staying over/ flirting on phone/ chatting on net) = fat thighs. Deal with it.	You don't need to listen to anybody just because they are older than you, but it helps to know their point of view. Learn to listen to yourself and to your reasonable self. Don't take decisions (big or small) when you are crying, angry, upset or laughing beyond control☺. Take them when you are calm. Get the information you need on sex, vagina, intercourse, porn from a reliable source (school counsellor/parent/sex education programme) and know that it's natural and not shameful to know about your body. How much of your sms-es/phone calls/ emails/clothes/body/ thoughts/ physical or emotional intimacy you want to share with your friends is your call. Having said that, these are not things that will buy you love or approval.

Real life diet analysis

Disha Arora is a fourteen-year-old school-going girl.

She feels she is overweight and, at fourteen, has already visited a number of dieticians in her attempt to lose weight.

She does not eat well because of the fear of putting on more weight, and has been told by elders around her that she needs to watch her weight and therefore watch her food! Disha's mother is also very unappreciative of Disha's body and often nags her about it. (When you have been brought up with this sort of conditioning and have been made to believe that being 'fat' is not acceptable, it affects every aspect of your well-being in the future.)

Disha gets tired easily, does not look forward to any recreational activities, and goes for her classes because she is 'supposed to go'. She also has irregular and painful periods, and a week before her periods she starts to feel dull, sleepy and lethargic (PMS).

Three-day diet recall

Time	Food/Drink	Activity Recall	Workout
Day 1			
6.45 a.m.		Woke up	
7.00 – 7.30 a.m.			Went for a walk
7.45 a.m.	2 slices of toast, 1 glass milk		
7.50 a.m.		Left for school	
10.30 a.m.	2 slices brown bread with garlic chutney		
	Did not have lunch because of a stomach ache		
3.15 p.m.		Reached home	
4.00 p.m.	2 slices of toast, egg white omelette, 1 glass milk		
4.30 – 5.00 p.m.		Rested	
5.20 – 6.30 p.m.	Had a fruit at 6 p.m.	Drawing class	
6.30 – 8.00 p.m.		Studied	
7.30 p.m.	1 roti, a bowl kadhi, ½ cup baingan, 3 small papads		
8.45 – 9.45 p.m.			Dance class
10.00 – 11.00 p.m.		Watched TV	

11.15 p.m.		Went to bed	
Day 2 (Holiday)			
6.50 a.m.		Woke up	
7.30 a.m.	2 slices of toast + 1 glass milk		
8.00 – 10.15 a.m.		Chemistry/biology tuitions	
10.30 a.m. – 1.00 p.m.		English tuitions	1 hour walking while studying
1.20 p.m.			Climbed stairs while going up
1.30 p.m.	2 besan parathas, 1 cup gravy aloo, ½ cup dahi		
1.30 – 3.00 p.m.		Rested, ate lunch, watched TV	
3.00 p.m.	2 small chocolates		
3.00 – 7.30 p.m.		Studied	
6.45 p.m.	1 bowl dry bhel		
7.30 – 8.30 p.m.		Watched TV, rested, got ready	
8.45 p.m.		Left for dinner	
9.30 p.m.	Dinner at a restaurant: 4 pieces fish, 1 piece chicken, 1 roti, 1 cup rice		
11.30 p.m.		Returned home	
12.45 a.m.		Went to bed; was reading before that	
Day 3			
7.00 a.m.		Woke up, got ready for school	
7.40 a.m.	Glass of milk		
7.45 a.m.		Left for school	

10.30 a.m.	1 egg white omelette		
1.00 p.m.	1 cup upma		
3.00 p.m.	1 bowl pangiri		
3.30– 4.30 p.m.		Rested, watched TV	
4.30 p.m.		Sat to study	
6.30 p.m.	2 cups rice, 1 bowl dal, 3 small papads		
9.00 – 10.00 p.m.		Watched TV	
11.00 p.m.		Went to sleep	

Evaluation of the recall

From her recall, you can see that Disha is making attempts to 'lose weight' — she exercises whenever she gets the time; she also takes the stairs, thinking that this will help her lose weight!

She does a lot of things through the day: school, tuitions, classes, exercise. But she is not eating nutritionally adequate food to sustain her. At this age, she needs to ensure that her body has all the nutrients it needs — the right proportion of carbs, protein, fat along with all other essential vitamins and minerals.

Once her body has the right nutrients and she exercises regularly, her lean body weight (muscle and bone weight) will increase, which will ensure stronger bones. (During adolescence, the body forms about half the bone mass it will ever have.) Also, as her lean body weight increases, her fat burning process will also improve (as muscle is the only metabolically active tissue in the body).

It is important for young kids, especially girls, to develop an admiration for their bodies and love their bodies for what they are. Constant nagging from family members (which is something young girls are vulnerable to), creates a feeling of hatred towards their bodies — eventually leading to fat storage. The more the body feels loved at this age, the more you will look good and you won't store any fat.

To look good, we first need to feel good from within! Disha just needed this — the 'feel good' factor.

The minute she would start loving her body, appreciating it and eating right (especially the foods she loved but avoided because of constant nagging), her nutrient absorption and assimilation would improve, her body cells would feel happier, her hormones would feel more privileged, her skin would glow like never before, her energy levels would soar high and her body fat levels would drop!

Modifications

Disha needed to eat frequent meals through the day. She just needed to nourish her growing body cells, and not compromise on her favourite foods — cheese, banana, suji halwa, paneer, pasta. Yummy ☺.

The diet recommended for Disha was as below:

Meal 1 (7.00 a.m.): Glass of milk

Meal 2 (8.00 a.m.): Banana

Meal 3 (10.30 a.m.): 2 egg whites + 2 slices whole wheat toast or suji halwa (something she loves, but used to avoid, thinking it's fattening!)

Meal 4 (1.00 p.m.): Roti + sabzi

Meal 5 (3.30 p.m.): Chicken breast + roti or homemade pasta with veggies

Meal 6 (5.30 p.m.): Cheese/soy milk

Meal 7 (7.30 p.m.): Roti + paneer sabzi

Meal 8 (9.00 p.m.): Glass of chaas

As Disha started eating nutritionally adequate foods, she started feeling much more energetic through the day. She started enjoying her exercise and would look forward to it, rather than being pushed into it.

She also started sleeping early and she would wake up fresh and energetic (and not lethargic). She was able to concentrate better on her studies as well, because of all these changes.

She was excited about the fact that she was eating all her favourite foods and was still losing weight (fat), and the words 'PMS', 'period cramps' and 'sweet cravings' were history for Disha!

Although her mother felt she needed to work more at losing weight, Disha was extremely happy with the changes that were taking place in her body and how good and comfortable she felt with her body now, so the nagging didn't bother her at all.

Disha has now developed an unconditional love for her body, which is surely going to take her a long way in her journey to achieve a fit and healthy body!

3

Marriage: Learning To Be

Real life example

'Come on, you are looking fab.... You don't think so?'
Monica sat unmoved. 'Come on, it's the first time I'm
seeing you in a short, sleeveless T-shirt.'

Some movement. 'Ya, I could never have imagined that
I would ever, *ever* be able to wear a sleeveless T-shirt.'

Monica had been on the diet plan with me for almost
six months now (including a few breaks/shaadis/holidays
and all of the usual stuff in between, but more or less 'at
it' for six months). The stretch marks on her arms had
gone and she had lost six kilos, dropped two sizes in jeans
(now wore a thirty-two-inch waist, and not to forget the
sleeveless Ts as well), could do five kilometres in thirty
minutes on the treadmill and thirty surya namaskars
(up from five kilometres in fifty minutes minimum, and
barely three or four surya namaskars) — all brilliant
changes, and all in a super short time according to me.
Not according to her. Monica felt she had done terribly,
and that I had let her down because there was 'just no
weight loss'.

'I know all that jazz about my looking better than ever,
no stretch marks, and I have so much more stamina. But
I want weight loss now. Bas! I don't want to listen to any
more jazz about my lean body weight going up or bone
getting denser and stuff.'

'Really? You know what your best friend went through, right?'

'Ya, but I'm not asking for anything that fast. Her results were so good that nazar to lagni thi!'

For the record, her best friend had gotten 'amazing results' — seventeen kilos lost in two months from being on a crash diet. Then one day, as she hit the brakes of her car, she felt something pop in her vagina. She was rushed to a hospital where the gynaecologist informed her that it was her uterus collapsing. The 'diet' had killed all the abdominal muscles necessary to hold the uterus in place. 'Are you actually saying this?' I asked Monica, incredulous.

'Yes, my weight loss is SO SLOOOW. One kilo a month! I have no face left. My parents have wasted so much money on all this weight loss, diets, exercise — what do I tell them? I am running faster on the treadmill so it's all okay? I need to be at least fifty-eight kilos.'

'Monica, give yourself some more time and you will be under fifty-five kilos if you are persistent.'

'When? Ten years later? I'm twenty-eight, damn it. Unmarried! Once I cross thirty, nobody will want to touch me (read I will lose all prospects in the marriage market), phir mein bhagti rahungi treadmill pe, getting nowhere in life, killing my time with hundred-two hundred surya namaskars.'

'You are so stressed. Ultimately your parents want you to marry because they want to see you happy. You will be happy if you find a guy who loves, supports and accepts you the way you are. Not because you are five kilos lighter.'

'Sheesh ... You will never understand what it means to be a marriageable girl from a rich Marwari family in south Mumbai.'

I shouldn't have, because I was a middle-class Marathi mulgi from Andheri. But I did. Because Virar to Vashi, Kashmir to Kanyakumari, this was one problem everybody understood, irrespective of caste, class, creed, religion. The 'thin, fair, tall' and preferably convent-educated phenomenon. We all understand this, we all really do. It binds our men together (more than cricket, even), they all want the same girl. And all girls want to be her even if it means killing who they are.

Jeans versus genes

The jeans you find in stores are not tailor-made for your body, so please, don't try and tailor-make your body to fit those jeans. If you feel bad that the jeans you're trying on fit your hips but not your waist, or vice versa, don't kill yourself over it. Just try another brand. And if no brand really fits, don't wear jeans. Or get a pair made for yourself. It's absolutely normal if a particular pair of jeans can't be pulled up beyond your thighs, or doesn't fit your hips — *it wasn't made for you.* A T-shirt is easier to fit into because it doesn't move through so many joints. A pair of pants has to move past your knees and hips — two major joints.

I know women who are so desperate to fit into a pair of jeans, they will lie down on their bed so they can zip up and button their pants. If you're so desperate that you'll stuff yourself into a pair of pants, you don't just risk looking odd (yes, it *is* evident to everyone that you've forced yourself into those pants), you're practically forcing your vagina to develop an infection because there's no air circulation.

People say that Indians are genetically bigger on the hips like there's something wrong with that. There's nothing wrong: just stop trying to fit into some standard-sized pair of jeans.

The thin, fair, tall and convent-educated phenomenon

Why did Monica want to be at least fifty-eight kilos? So that she could write fifty-five kilos on her bio data for the marriage bureau. Yes, that has to be included compulsorily. So, along with your age, height, colour of the skin, birth date and time, you have to fill up the weight category too, and then of course attach a picture. Some bureaus are strict and will ask for one full-length and one close-up picture. For Monica, writing fifty-five while her weight was still around sixty-three didn't seem right.

I could understand what she was going through, but felt very strongly that she was in a position where she could stand up for herself instead of complying with the norms. To be fair, she had often tried. All the lines that she had given to me earlier 'after I cross thirty, nobody will want to touch me … blah blah' were her mother's copyrighted responses when Monica would suggest that the diet plan with me was working because she no longer had food cravings, her stretch marks were disappearing and she felt stronger and more energetic — though, of course, the numbers on the scale didn't say all this about her.

Her mother had strongly opposed her decision to study finance in the UK, and had predicted that it would be difficult to get a groom if she studied 'too much'. In her mom's opinion, she should have stayed back in Mumbai, helped dad or chacha/mama types with their accounts, taken some cooking classes (even salsa and Pilates if she wanted), generally hung around so that they could start 'looking', and by twenty-three/twenty-four, be married. As a reward, her mom was ready to sponsor a trip to Switzerland (like Kajol in DDLJ) for her and her cousin. Monica now felt that it was a rocking plan, but at that time she had 'finance ka bhoot' and her dad had relented and thought it was alright to let her pursue the one-year diploma.

That one year had gotten her five kilos heavier. She had stayed back for two more years to work in a UK firm after getting an on-campus offer. Finally the family put their foot down and Monica moved back home some ten kilos heavier than when she'd left and angry at the diktat of being told to move back with no concern for her career. But at least, she thought, she would be home, and it would be okay since there were so many MNCs now. To her dismay, she hardly felt at home in the house she'd grown up in; in three years a lot seemed to have changed somehow.

Her family now actively started 'looking'. She put her job-hunt on hold because she thought it would be better to find work according to where she would live after marriage. Her family decided she should lose some weight to better her chances of getting married, so she had gone from one fad diet to another, losing some weight, gaining back some more, and in the process upsetting her menstrual cycle, skin, hair and developing stretch marks in the bargain.

She soon removed conditions like 'boy should be from Mumbai', 'family should be okay with me working', etc. and made it easier for herself and her family to turn her into a non-entity that had to be married. In the process of becoming less of a problem for her family, she had turned out to be the biggest problem for herself. She could no longer identify with the person she had become. Her daily activities like helping in the kitchen, losing weight, looking good, meeting boys under parental guidance, etc. were not challenging enough for her intelligence. Her confidence was super low with all the rejections she had received from men who inspired no respect, no 'ting ting' in the heart, nothing, and yet she desperately wished that one of them would say 'yes' and she could escape from this 'hell' that she created for herself and from what she had become.

Uff! It's just too complicated but we all understand this. We truly do. Either we have been one of Monica's kind — a bright spark (too bright to marry quickly and settle down or too bright that you unintentionally unnerve the prospective groom or too independent that the groom's family decides that you can't adjust to their ways and customs, even when you have almost killed yourself proving that you will, in fact you have!) — or know more than one girl who shares a similar story. What is understandable — actually not really, perhaps I should word it like this — what needs to change is how the Monicas of this world respond to this predicament. Perhaps they should start putting their foot down and follow their heart — whether the heart takes them to another job, another land, another family, whatever. And then they should take the consequences of following their heart in their stride instead of feeling guilty or ashamed about their intelligence and independent bent of mind. As a society we should support all women we know in choosing their paths and guide them into being their own person instead of all of us trying to be exactly like each other, or desperately trying to fit into a mould.

After all we owe our lives, freedom, education to all the nameless, faceless women who pursued education, art, wore pants, had careers, stepped outside of family domains to create their own worlds and chose to face being ostracised by society or get labelled as 'modern', 'chalu', 'fast', etc. to be their own people, for choosing to not wear masks, for choosing to live with dignity and self-respect. Please note that when men do the unconventional, they become heroes and leaders; women simply get labels. If our lives are better today, if we take education for granted today (a lot of women in our country can't read; irrespective of whether you like or dislike this book, you're amongst the lucky few who can read, have money to buy books and the luxury of worrying about body weight); if we don't get labelled for pursuing art, literature, a career in armed forces, or travel alone, live alone, make money, etc. it's all thanks to the sacrifices of women who changed society to make this acceptable. Empowered women who are free to make decisions for themselves are happier and it leads to a peaceful and happy society. When women are constantly under threat or suppressed, the entire society suffers. Just look at Afghanistan.

Marriage: All eggs in one basket?
And seriously, what else other than our own limitations and confusion is coming in the way of leading life to its fullest. Monica had spent years — from when she was twenty-four to twenty-eight, the prime of her youth — being somebody else (marriageable), someone

she couldn't relate to. In the process she had become so bitter about herself that she oozed frustration and anger. These are typically the women about whom we crack smart alec jokes like, 'She just needs to get laid, man'. Monica was not sure if she wanted to get married at this cost (boy, it had taken a toll on her health) and yet she was guilty that she had gone against her parents' wishes and was ready to compensate by 'at least now' doing what they wanted her to do. During this guilt trip she had forgotten that she should have anticipated the consequences of what she was doing to herself or made five/ten-year projections, like they had taught her at finance school. If the projections were not in line with the investments, then the investments needed to be altered.

A sensible finance professional never puts money in NPA (non-performing assets). Also a sensible finance person, and for that matter even a non-finance person, knows the thumb rule for investments — 'Never put all your eggs in one basket'. Then how come we overlook this when we invest all our time, money, effort, emotions, all our resources in the one singular basket of marriage? Just like a diversified portfolio leads to a stable and healthy financial life, diversified investments in all aspects of our life — art, culture, education, health, freedom, companionship, charity, career, etc. will lead to a stable and healthy state of mind and body.

When you put all your eggs in one basket it's called gambling. Ghoda chal gaya to chal gaya nahi to raste pe aaoge. So **it's really unfair for the institution of marriage itself that we peg all our hope, happiness**

and sense of stability and security on just this one thing. In fact, all that this does is make marriage difficult, uninteresting, suffocating and boring. For marriage to be fulfilling, peaceful and everlasting, both the partners should have strength, stability and flexibility to let the partner be. It's like a trikonasana — your pose will be perfect when both your right and left sides do what they are meant to do without wavering or being unduly influenced by the other. So when you extend and bend to the right, the rotation on your waist, the flexibility in your hip and the reach of your arm depends on how steady, strong and stable the left leg, hip, chest, shoulder and arm is. If the centre of your body, the navel, responsible for maintaining equilibrium, moves to the right or to the dominant side, then the pose is lost. So for the navel to stay in the centre you need a left side which does its job well and doesn't move to the right; it also ensures that you will actually get a good extension on the right. Now you have a good pose.

Similarly, in a marriage the woman should have the inner peace, strength and wisdom to do her part to the fullest, only then can the marriage remain stable and happy. If you are constantly dominated by your husband or peg all your hopes on him, you are not just ruining your own growth, but also his.

I think that's enough gyaan about why women should invest in a diversified way in their life and not hope that marriage will fulfil all their needs and wants, including physical, emotional, mental and spiritual. Marriage can be one of the things that fulfil you, but not the *only* thing.

So Monica should have still remained interested and invested in getting a good workout, studying, working, travelling because she found fulfilment and excitement in all these things instead of just shaadi. It rhymes with barbadi!

Trousseau thin

My inbox is loaded with emails saying, 'I'm getting married in two months and I want to lose weight. It's my day and I really want to look great.' Hello, you shouldn't think that you need to get fit only because you're getting all this designer stuff from Kolkata, Delhi, etc. Do you really want to be 'trousseau thin', fitting into those fabulous clothes only at the wedding, and wanting to jump out the window every time you look at them after that? If you want to be thin, then it should be a lifelong commitment, not for ten days before and ten days after the event. And another thing — what is the whole 'I want to lose weight to get married' drama. No man in his right frame of mind will accept or reject a woman based on her size. If he does, then, believe me, you don't want to be with him. There need to be more solid reasons for you'll to stay together. A sensible partner is only interested in your staying healthy and fit, calm and comfortable with your body. All of us want to be with a guy with his head on his shoulders, not a guy who judges us.

Pre-marriage weight loss

Your desire to lose weight should be to get healthier and stronger in the body and to reach a level of fitness that makes it easier to go after all your pursuits towards excellence and a meaningful existence. Anyway, let's look at why we are so obsessed with weight loss for marriage! There are largely two reasons for this: the evolutionary reason and the conditional response or internalised social or cultural response.

Waist to hip ratio – the evolutionary reason
Let's look at the evolutionary reason. During
would you prefer a leaner partner? By the way, even men
try to lose weight for the wedding day, though of course
the pressure on them is much less. And if they are good at
what they do, come from a good family background and
earn well, they don't need to be lean or muscular. But if
you belong to the female gender, then even though you
might meet all the other criteria, you will also need to be
thin and fair; we can relax on the 'tall' bit.

Okay, getting to the point, heard of the waist-to-hip
ratio? Measure the narrowest part of your waist, just a
little above your navel, and then the broadest part of your
hips. Now divide your waist size by your hip size. What's
the figure? If it's 0.7, well you make a good mate (not
to be confused with the Australian 'mate'). The waist-
to-hip ratio, among many other things, is an indicator
of fitness, fertility, strength and yeah, beauty too. (The
optimum ratio for men is 0.9.) Therefore, irrespective
of your body weight and waist measurement, whether
you wear a twenty-six, thirty, thirty-six, or can't fit into
ready-made jeans at all, as long as you are in proportion,
you fit the bill. In case of climatic change, flood, famine,
food shortage, etc., you will survive, give birth to
healthier off-spring with improved chances of survival
and the process of evolution will love you because you
are fit to carry its work forward. This is found across
cultures and is rooted deep in the selection process for
mating (and marriage is seeking community or social
acceptance of the mating process). So, though African
women differ in size and shape from the European or

the petite oriental women, the ones with a ratio closer to 0.7 will be preferred as partners to mate with. African women will have big hips and big waists, and Southeast Asians will have a small hip bone and a tiny waist to go with it.

You could be petite, medium-framed or broad-built, as long as you maintain optimum body fat levels, your waist and hip will be in proportion to each other. The waist will be the narrowest part of the midriff with no fat hanging around it, and the hips will be full and round and the largest part. This proportion gives insight into your menstrual cycle and therefore hormonal harmony or balance. Women who take good care of themselves, not just in terms of food and exercise, but also in terms of overall growth, challenge their mental limitations/conditioning, indulge in creative pursuits and take ownership of their life and all the ups and downs that come with it, generally maintain good fitness levels. Their body fat levels are never abnormally high or low, so their hormones are in a good place. This helps them maintain a healthy metabolic rate, ovulation, immunity levels, skin, hair and nails as well.

The ratio is also an indicator of fat distribution, especially the visceral fat. Visceral fat is the fat that you collect on the abdomen. Subcutaneous fat is the fat we carry all over the body under our skin. **From a pure health perspective (and now also from the perspective of attractiveness), it's better to have less fat deposits around the viscera or stomach area and have your fat distributed all over your body.** This is only possible when you eat right and work out. So we should stop this mad rush to lose weight and look to achieving healthier body fat levels and improve on health parameters. Work out and eat right so that the fat is well distributed and not just loaded at one place. You must have often noticed that women with PCOS/PCOD have waists that balloon out of the body. PCOS/PCOD can lead to insulin insensitivity and a host of other issues including infertility in the long term, and is mostly a result of a poor lifestyle, inactivity and processed food (see Chapter 6). So while they have these problems, they can never fit into the optimum waist-to-hip ratio.

Also, if you have gone through a crash diet which doesn't promote eating right and regular exercise, or signed up for one of those 'pay for ten kilos, lose five kilos free', or the ones which promise weight loss even though you stay immobile, 'no exercise, no sweat' types, then you will have a lowered body weight (only for a while though), but also a flatter butt and love handles around your waist, and again you won't get the optimum waist-hip ratio, and therefore not the goodness that optimum body fat can bring to life. Needless to say, your menstrual cycle, hormones, bone density, metabolic rate, skin, hair and nails will all be upset at being put through this unnecessary torture of 'weight loss'.

Think about it, if bureaus (and now websites) ask for your waist-to-hip ratio, they are actually being discreet. You won't need to put your weight down or your vital stats; this also ensures that there will be less cheating. Because a figure like 0.7 or 0.8 etc. will give away nothing other than the status of your health. It will also prevent a lot of young women from almost killing themselves (literally and figuratively) over losing weight.

Conditional response
So from the evolutionary point of view it makes sense to want to get leaner for the mating process (doesn't make sense to lose weight though) and increase chances of healthier progeny. The other cultural or learned social responses are a little more complicated. For one, marriages are not gender neutral. I mean, if you are a son-in-law, what your in-laws expect of you is completely different from what in-laws expect from a daughter-in-law. Let's say you are a girl who is now married and are answering an sms on your phone while your MiL/FiL is talking to you. If they don't get upset with you for that harmless activity or assume that this amounts to indifference/disrespect, then they are worth preserving as the rare species of 'progressive/understanding in-laws'. If you are a son-in-law, then you don't see any reason to preserve them; I mean, come on, though you were wildly sms-ing you were also listening very attentively, you even looked up once and asked if there's some more gajar halwa. Anyways, to understand the concept of conditional response better, try out this experiment.

Fitting in

I have always felt getting married makes a girl's position akin to that of an average Indian tourist in, say, Rishikesh, Goa or Dharamsala. You are better than the average gora, have more money, don't bargain as much as the Israeli, are friendlier than the American, less demanding than the

French, don't smoke as much as the Italian but the locals or the hotel/shack/shop owners don't seem to want you. They prefer the gora. You can sense it; you may enjoy the place, but you start feeling the discrimination as soon as you make 'grih pravesh'. You find yourself making senseless efforts to fit in or to become more acceptable. You dress in clothes you wouldn't normally wear, eat organic salad and yak cheese even if you don't like the taste, and wear slippers that are clearly not going to last you for more than a week.

You don't need to, but you desperately try to fit in and try to woo the locals even you don't know for what. And honestly, your stupid or jhalla behaviour has more to do with your own bias or inferiority complex. Slowly but surely you come to realise that you are discriminating against yourself much more than the locals. You don't have to wear harem pants and a T-shirt with Krishna playing his flute just because you are in Rishikesh, or tiny shorts with a spaghetti top just because you are in Goa. Similarly, you don't have to be thin just because you want to get married. I think this get thin for marriage is majorly wanna-be behaviour, just like most other things associated with it.

An experiment — peeche se pressure

Travel in a Virar local, preferably the fast 12 coach. As you squeeze yourself in and feel suffocated or think this is probably how you will feel when you are taking the last few breaths of your life, the woman in front says, 'Kiti praishure', and you will retort, 'Main kya karu, peeche se kitna pressure hai!' It's the same thing with shaadi, peeche se kitna pressure. So if you want to do what the Mahatma said, be the change you want to see, you've got to be strong and flexible, bearing all the load that's coming from behind (tradition, culture, religion, family, etc.), protecting your organs from getting contorted in the journey and also the lady in front who can then breathe free because your weight is no longer pushing her down or out of the train. If you are not strong enough to bear the weight of this suffocating journey, then you will only pass on the burden ahead, harming the woman in front and in the process harming your organic body, and feel further suffocated and claustrophobic.

So look at the women who board the fast train: they stand prepared with the resolve and focus of Usain Bolt at the start line, and look at how well they equip themselves. The dupattas come to the front and no longer stylishly sway on the butt, the saree pallu goes deep inside the creases of the saree, damn the ironing, the younger ones wear their backpacks on the chest, clip their hair, change into flat chappals and board that train, ready to deal with the pressure both aage se and peeche se. And guess what, a good enough percentage of these women actually enjoy or in fact look forward to making this journey daily. The only thing that makes them capable of enjoying these almost inhuman conditions is that they understand what the pressures are and equip themselves to deal with it, and strike friendship with other strong women who have learnt to deal with it as well. The unrelenting Mumbai spirit? Or a lesson in holding your ground and enjoying the glorious journey called marriage?

That we should get fitter, leaner, stronger because it's good for our own health and peace of mind is totally relevant. That we want or are intrinsically attracted to leaner and fitter partners from an evolution point of view also makes sense. **But that we 'must lose weight' to get married is only peeche ka pressure.** Equip yourself to deal with it, don't get swayed by that demand. Or else we will only turn into those irritating women who will eventually stress their daughters, nieces, neighbour's daughter, daughter-in-law, granddaughter, sis-in-law and basically all of womankind to 'lose weight for shaadi'. Surely you don't want to turn into one of them.

Marriage turns the most accomplished, talented, beautiful, self-assured girl into a second-class citizen. The first right over resources — dinner, the side of the bed, TV programme, glass of chaas — anything at all belongs to the husband. And it takes time for even the most self-assured or self-respecting girl to stop discriminating against herself or to create and unabashedly enjoy equality with her husband, be it sharing responsibilities or resources or recreation. So all in all it takes a while and some introspection for most girls to start being themselves or else they just try to be more acceptable, more lovable or more whatever and in that process lose their real selves. It's not uncommon to hear things like, 'Grow your hair now, the hairstyle will look better', or 'Try the entire body bleach or get the bikini wax done', or 'Do the special facials so that on the wedding day your face is glowing'. The point I am trying to make is that, big or small, harmless or harsh, there are numerous ways in which we as a society or individuals express just one thing — that as women we are inadequate. That weight loss, skin package, body bleach, threading (not to forget hymen reconstruction) will make us more deserving of the medal of husband/family that we're marrying into. This aspect needs to be understood better so that we don't harm our bodies and minds by some quick-fix therapies/diets/workouts, etc.

Flyovers

They are strong and are built to take the load of moving cars, trucks, etc. and the various forces they exert. If you ever stand on a flyover when the traffic is moving, you will feel it moving under your feet. That's the in-built flexibility of the flyover: the ability of the bridge to expand or stretch while there is traffic running over it. If it's too flexible it will never be strong enough to bear the weight, if it's too rigid, it will never be flexible enough to stand on its own under constantly changing loads and pressures. Marriage as an institution will break if it doesn't expand or change with changing times. Even today it's almost too rigid with the roles that men and women are supposed to play. If it has to survive, then it needs to bend, stretch, move, re-adjust to changing times and to the ever-evolving women species. Or else it will be lost just like the other close-to-extinction 'joint family system'.

Single in the city

There was a time when young women left their mothers' homes only when they got married, but that's changing these days. Now women move out either because they're working or studying in a different city.

Personally, I can make out women who've spent a lot of time in a hostel: there are less nutrients in the food so the women tend to have more problems with their hormones than those who've spent all their time at home. The latter almost always got fresh food — even if it was karela sabzi and they hated it — every day; it wasn't made two days ago, and for everyone in the building. So women in hostels have a compromised nutrient intake and absorption. They tend to put on weight not because of calories but largely because they didn't get enough nutrients in their growing years.

So when you decide to go to a hostel to study, the enthu with which you plan your hostel life, clothes, new sim card, phone, online connectivity, toiletries, how to keep in touch with bf, etc. plan for food as well. Look for some aunty who will deliver home-cooked dabbas, get a budget allotted for dry fruits, fruits and nuts, try and get an electric cooker and learn to make khichdi or aloo sabzi. It's not like a rule that everybody who goes to hostel will lose or gain five kilos in a year depending on how their body copes with loss of lean body weight. Haan, yes, also budget for and sincerely go to a gym/yoga class/swimming, whatever your calling. If you are a parent sending your daughter out, tell her in no uncertain terms that, less than five workouts a week, or less than twelve clean meals and she comes back home. Okay, that she doesn't get her new iPhone. Education or career should make us smart, not dull or fat.

Basically plan for eating good food and for exercising just like you plan for other things, keeping fit is just as important as education or career, it's not like you need to give up on one to get another.

Women who move out on their own usually share apartments and they don't invest in, or think it's uncool to invest in, setting up a working kitchen. Their kitchens are largely used just to make chai-coffee and include a microwave to heat up the leftovers from last night's take-away. So they just eat in their office canteens, or eat fast food. Little wonder that they put on weight and also have issues with their menstruation, cramps, bad skin, etc.

You have to understand that your hormones must always be in a state of balance — only then can you enjoy good health. If you lose this harmony, you'll see its loss reflected in your body, mind, etc. You've invested so much time and energy in finding an apartment. Now spend as much energy in getting a gas connection and kitchen utensils within a week of moving in. If you think you're too cool to cook, at least we're lucky to live in a country where it's easy to get someone to come home and do it for you. That way, you can be cool for a long time, not just be cool in your early twenties and then start looking like an aunty when you're twenty-four. That's right — **inadequate nutrients and not enough antioxidants will lead to too much of the free radical effect and therefore a quicker ageing process.**

The emerging single woman

More and more women today are giving up on the traditional dictum of compromise. And it's not just that they've figured out that they don't want to compromise on the guy — they don't want to compromise themselves and what they believe in. We're finally seeing the reality that it's not just about hooking up with a guy, so a lot of women are choosing to stay single. As part of a larger community of women, we should all support this, not wonder what's wrong, or try and set up your single friend with someone she'll never get along with or your cousin in New Jersey who's looking to 'settle'.

A woman who's single has that much more to do and take care of: plumbing, get the car serviced, attend the building general body meeting, so she tends to feel like there's little time to exercise. I tend to hear these same old excuses: either my client has a husband to take care of and that's why she has no time to exercise, or she's single and she has so many things to take care of so she has no time. If you're single, and think you're smarter than what's available, then be smart and make the time to exercise. We're so used to supporting a child, an ailing father, etc. that we don't stop to think about the support *we* need, nutritionally, emotionally. There's an unacknowledged battle for acceptance that single women face — did you know that a single woman with a 10 lakh rupee income will get a smaller loan than a married woman with a 10 lakh rupee income? — and they may sometimes feel very upset, start questioning themselves, and one of the things that suffers is food.

As a single woman, you are braving so many things: you should understand that if you want a strong mind, you need a strong body.

Post-marriage weight gain

Post marriage everybody gains weight, both men and women, but somehow it's much more apparent in women. Oh why oh why oh why? Again, a bit of it is peeche se pressure, but come on, we can't blame everything on pressure, so let's look at what happens post shaadi which makes it easy for us to gain weight and difficult for us to fit into those relaxed-fit Esprit jeans. Ah ha, we are now having sex. Yeah, you've heard that before. Sillies, there are enough marriages out there where partners haven't touched each other in days/months/years. Also, there are enough out there who have been sexually active before getting hitched. So this shaadi and sex theory is too flawed for any discussion. Then how come both these extremes and everybody in between is gaining weight?

Sex and weight

If anything, a healthy sex life makes you leaner and fitter by helping you relax, unwind and rejoice. So a good sex life leads to better physical health and mental well-being and no, it doesn't make your weight increase! And I think it's our sick mind at play again, the thing that the glossies, gossip papers and Mrs Sharma told you. If you enjoy something then it must be fattening. Get off it. Bananas, mangoes, chole puri, gulab jamun, the chutney with the idli, the coconut in your curry, the ghee on your khichdi and sex are NOT fattening. Remember, if you are enjoying it, it will burn fat for you.

After marriage, women are conditioned to not just give up their name (maiden name — yeh kya term hai? Why no bachelor/boy name for men?), home and hearth, but also other things that are intrinsic to our core: food, meal-size, meal-timings (gym and yoga teacher too, if you change cities or even localities). Now since you go to the boy's house (no, they are not men yet; they are Mummyji's li'l boys), well you are expected to change. Please don't ask where this expectation comes from — it's years of regression, suppression, peeche se pressure, andar se pressure and a bit of mindless compliance, lack of clarity, affirmation and obviously self-esteem which leads to this 'let me walk all over myself to win your approval and get into your good books' attitude.

All these changes (and more) manifest themselves as 'weight gain'. Here's how:

1. Your meal times change.

And so do your vitamin B stores. The first few days your meal timings change because of shaadi and functions pre and post. You are not just eating meals cooked for hajjar people, but also at really weird times. None of the rules of increasing nutrient absorption are being followed (see Introduction). You are simply busy looking like a million bucks on the outside while your intestines are almost rotting with all the toxins caused by over-eating, mithai and atrocious meal timings; the hormones are all over the place; the enzymes are feeling punished — and there you are, standing and smiling for pictures.

Just as you are recovering from the shaadi, you go for your honeymoon, which again involves more eating out, travelling (the richer you are — or your parents are — the more you travel), so from Lonavala to London, Goa to Guantanamo (oh! is that a torture cell?), you travel, eat on flights/trains/buses, eat packaged food and 'enjoy' yourself with wine, pastry, cakes, etc. The poor stomach is surely against big weddings and honeymoons, whether or not you are. No wonder it's called the big FAT wedding — it surely makes you fat, and how! So though you did 'nothing' and 'relaxed' during your honeymoon, you still come back home dead tired, so tired that you almost feel like you need a honeymoon to recover from your honeymoon.

Think hard about why this happens. Primarily two reasons: you are just too tired digesting all the food you have dabaoed over the last fifteen-twenty days, and the mind is drained with all the anxiety and stress of the shaadi, naya ghar, etc. The stress of such a big function (which everybody will dissect and comment about) and all the food and all the late nights take a toll on the most primary and energy-giving vitamin of your body — vitamin B. (It has no calories of its own but makes it easier for your body to metabolise your calories, especially the ones that come from carbs, which every Indian wedding feast is rich in.)

Some of the ways a vitamin B deficiency will manifest are:

- A strong urge to sleep every morning even if you have slept for a full eight hours.
- Constipation and bloating.
- Mood swings and going into full senti mode for no reason at all.

- Feeling like you are in some trance or feeling like doing nothing.
- Wanting to go to mummy's house, now!

If you felt all these immediately after the shaadi till the time you thought that you will probably feel exactly like this all your life so you just stopped noticing it, then you are guilty of stretching yourself more than you are capable of or have the strength to bear. One of the main changes with getting married, whether you stay with just the husband or with all the other paraphernalia, is the toll that it takes on your meal timings. You have to just adapt to the timings of your 'family' or learn to eat at a time that is convenient to your bai or come home and cook depending on what time you got back, how much energy you have to cook, is there a vegetable at all in the fridge or will you now need to go down and refill your oil/salt ka dabba, or what time your husband comes home! So while you cope with the new family, dhobi, mali, corner shop, etc., you forget that for years together you are used to or like eating at a certain time.

Not eating at the right time leads to overeating at weird hours, which drains your intestines of all the essential flora, B vitamins and healthy bacteria. Little wonder then that, both physically and mentally, you feel 'not quite up to it', dull, or just overwhelmed by changes, not just in how you are supposed to behave, talk, feel as a married woman (the driver and bhaji wala start calling you bhabhi, the building kids may contribute to your grief by calling you aunty), but of those that happen in your own body. Slowly the waist circumference increases, the lower abdomen starts bulging and the navel starts moving away from the spine. The body starts ageing almost abruptly; it's a bit of a paradox — like feeling lonely in a mehfil.

And calcium goes too: Carbs, proteins and fats are metabolised by B vitamins; a lot of the 'feel good' factor in the brain is also because of B vitamins. Since your lifestyle changes in a way that you don't quite anticipate, there's a drop in vitamin B levels, which leads to the increased consumption of refined foods and sugars — stuff like shakes, pastries, mithai, chocolates, biscuits, breads, fries, farsan, sev, etc. (Look at any bhel puri wala — who do you find there in large numbers, young teenage girls or the married aunty types?) The increase in refined food consumption further depletes B vitamins, thus leading to the other big loss — that of calcium from the bones.

Most of my married women clients (especially after having kids) report needing a piece of chocolate or gulab jamun post a meal, especially post dinner (they take great pride in the fact that they never eat the entire bar, just one chintu little piece). This is nothing but a sign of depleted vitamin B and calcium along with a few other minerals like selenium and chromium caused by long gaps between meals followed by overeating, and an increased consumption of chai/coffee. Almost every girl drinks more caffeine in the 'husband's house' as compared to their 'mother's house'. Arrey, is it because we become homeless or is it a plain 'use a drug to cope up with life' strategy? After marriage, the foundation for the false belief 'I have a sweet tooth' starts taking root; it then grows into a full-fledged condition or deficiency usually after the birth of the second child or before your first child turns five or after you have gone through that pregnancy treatment for three to five years (depending on what is applicable to you). (The only thing that can make you susceptible to this condition pre-marriage is crash dieting or mindless gymming and exercise.)

Also what is it with eating chintu pieces of chocolate? Young, unmarried or teenage girls eat the entire bar and flash waists that look yummy; the married ones soon lose self-esteem and don't think that they deserve a full bar so they 'discipline and control' themselves and 'limit' themselves to one piece. Let's get real, one piece a day is far more dangerous than a bar a month or while on holiday. What's easier to cope with — your husband's constantly roving eye or one full-fledged affair?

And so do your sleep timings: As you eat later in the nights and sleep even later (your husband is not keeping you up, shy little girl, that's just filmy interpretation of restless nights), you wake up dead tired. Now if you are married into a joint family, then you will HAVE to wake up before the rest of the family and bathe and be ready and all that. Exaggerated? Okay, you will have to wake up at least before 8 a.m.? Waking up after that will earn you tags like 'lazy', 'aaj kal ki ladkiyan', 'mummy ne kuch sikhaya nahi' or you will be gently reminded that 'hamare ghar mein sab...', or 'hamari to himmat hi nahi hoti thi, zamana badal gaya hai chalo accha hai', or your sis-in-law grudgingly says that she wished she had the guts to do what you do. Hello! You just woke up an hour later at the most, and your husband — for the record — is still snoring. If you are not in a joint family, even then your MiL will graciously volunteer to stay back the first few days to guide you with the reet–rivaz of the house or ask you to stay with her for ten–fifteen days so that you can learn 'hamare tarike' and the bhindi ka bhaji that Pinku loves. Even if you have been spared the gracious volunteering, then you still have the job (you just got it, we don't need your CV; you are now an unpaid employee of what is supposed to be your home) of keeping your house running. So you wake up to the bai, dudhwalla, car-washing guy…. And lack of sleep, as I've mentioned before, causes damage to your hormones and metabolism (more in Chapter 7).

2. The way the bhindi is getting cut changes.
Changes in how the food is made, the masala used, oil, salt, the ginger in the chai — all of it further stresses your stomach and intestinal lining. At your mom's, you are used to a certain amount and style of cooking, so your stomach knows what to expect. When, all of a sudden, the taste, consistency, flavours change, the stomach doesn't quite understand what's happening. The intestines rebel a bit by changing your urinating and defecating patterns and hope that you will listen and go back to what it's most comfortable with — both in terms of time and actual food taste. But you are obviously in no mood to listen, you are now happily married.

A friend of mine once had her FiL in a fit of rage because he was terribly upset at the way the bhindi had been cut!! The daughter-in-law had unintentionally and almost mechanically cut, cooked, spiced and flavoured the bhindi (a rage with all of us in the gang) the way she used to at her mom's; this turned out to be different from the way her mother-in-law cooked it. Forget the cooking, at least learn to cut the bhindi 'properly', advised her FiL (free advice along with free food). My girl friend went red-faced in anger at the humiliation, but she is from a 'good family' so she didn't answer back. Instead she cribbed to all of us about how she wished she could stuff the FiL instead of the bhindi!

The way veggies and fruits are cut and cooked can help retain a lot of nutrients, but imposing your style of sabzi (along with all other things) on your bahu when you don't have the stomach for even one variation or when you choose to remain unadventurous with your food (Switzerland mein Gujju thali milega kya?) is, to put it mildly, regressive. I mean preference is one thing, imposition quite another.

This 'mummy ke yahan and hamare yahan' is so much part of our psyche, that often girls don't learn to cook till they marry. Kya fayda? Anyway, shaadi ke baad toh sab naye se seekhna padega, they reason. So the girl remains like a blank canvas on which the husband's family can paint their cooking (and everything else) style. But come on, cooking is a life-saving skill. We all should know (irrespective of gender) how to cook, irrespective of our marital status.

3. You are now eating out more than ever.
Noticed that? Starts from when you're courting and then just keeps going on, shaadi, honeymoon, dinner invites and then graduates to let's eat out if the bai has not come, you've had a bad day at work or fought with each other,

to escape from eating with the in-laws again or to just get away from home. No marks for guessing, but it's much more than your 'Miss' days. I mean, some moms will even tell their daughter, Eat out as much as you want with your husband after you are married, right now I don't want to take the responsibility of you getting home late and all that. Apne ghar jao aur jo chahiye karo.

Now, again, eating out often takes a toll on your body composition and bloating levels. The big problem with eating out is, no matter how expensive or exclusive the restaurant you ate at, it still doesn't lead to satisfaction. Most times you feel restless after eating; you either need to reach for a frizzy drink (worse, we choose the 'diet' option because we feel so guilty about consuming calories) or a pastry or at least a coffee. There is a strong need for a neurological kick, because the food failed to comfort or satisfy.

The other way we try and feel 'complete' after a meal while eating out is to simply eat more than usual, but all that it does is make you feel stuffed and dull. That light, energetic (mitahar) feeling that we all naturally look for after we eat becomes an elusive experience. Eating becomes an escape rather than an act of nourishing your body, mind, senses and soul. The other thing it becomes, is entertainment.

4. You are now entertaining and being entertained more than ever.
Eating for entertainment is downright boring and unimaginative, besides being harmful for health. There was a time when women would go to temples to socialise: a lot of our festival rituals and customs are testimony to

that. Even today, in Chiplun (that's my — and Dawood's — ajol; ajol in Marathi is the village where your mother's parents come from), we all go to the temple during festivals. The entire community meets in the temple, sings, dances and eats in praise of the lord. Yeah, and we do all those other things too: wear good clothes and catch up with the rest of the Chiplunkars. In modern times, coffee shops and restaurants are replacing temples; the lord here is consumerism. Dress up, greet, eat, eat, eat, finish with a dessert and drown it in wine.

In the temple, you dress the deity too, clean up the premises, sing bhajans, cook food with others in your community, offer it to god and to underprivileged sections, eat (the same food) and generally the attitude is of devotion or bhakti bhav. Ever felt bhakti while eating the fettuccine with olives and parmesan or dum aloo biryani or chicken kebabs? Unlikely. You probably felt like a bhogi (opposite of yogi). A bhogi only cares about enjoying sensory pleasures; a yogi cares about going beyond the sensory pleasures and making every moment worthwhile. So eat out, entertain, get entertained and if you find meaning in it, your mind and body will be nourished by the vibes and the calories around. If it's purely an escape from boredom or depressing thoughts or one of those 'have to be seen there' things, then it's going to lead to dullness in both the mind and body. **A dull body, by the way, is the one which stores more than optimum levels of fat** (so again, you could weigh forty-five kilos or less, but if more than twenty-five per cent of your body weight comes from fat, you will feel dull).

If you find yourself meeting the girls for lunch/ coffee, meeting friends for dinner and drowning in beer, arranging mummyji's kitty lunch, little baby's fourth budday party with a theme and food that match and that romantic date with hubby is reduced to a late-night movie followed by dinner, or worse, TV and call the pizza guy, then trust me, you are doomed to stay fat. Find better ways of entertainment now! As a policy, avoid shopping and eating for entertainment.

The undercover gharwali

'I do nothing, I am a housewife' to the recent 'I am a homemaker': both statements mean that the woman is slogging at home, pursuing housework with the dedication one gives a career but not getting paid for it. And what about 'working' or 'career-oriented' women? Does working or pursuing your career make you a 'homebreaker' or 'workwife'? Personally, I hate labels (more than Rajesh Khanna hates tears). It's unfair to assume that a 'homemaker' doesn't have any ambition or will not develop one outside of her home duties or that a career-oriented woman gives a damn for how well her kitchen and home runs. In fact most of the times, women who work (in offices) slog doubly hard at home, they just don't get recognised for it. Preity Zinta, the bubbliest person I have worked with, wears many a hat: successful actor, successful business woman, UN goodwill ambassador, guardian to thirty-four girls in a school near Rishikesh, etc. She is good at all domesticated work (in her own words) but is best at cooking and takes keen interest in running an efficient kitchen and home (with her mom's help). She jokingly calls herself 'the undercover gharwali' because she realises that she may be known/acknowledged/awarded for all her work except for that which she puts in at home, but that doesn't reduce her interest or commitment towards it.

Isn't it high time our work at home becomes visible to us — eventually the housewife and the working woman both consider their work at home or their contribution towards home as 'nothing' and both feel guilty of not doing enough. God! I do hate labels except the 'undercover gharwali' ;-).

5. *You have now accepted that your husband/family/ Ramu kaka/Gangu bai/a clean bedroom/an efficiently-run kitchen (not necessarily in this order) are more important than you.*

'Why is there such a big gap between Meal 1 and Meal 2?' I asked Nisha.

'Arrey, time nahi milta between 8 and 11 a.m.,' she replied.

Nisha did all the usual things in the morning: organised breakfast, gave FiL his insulin, sent the kid off to school, instructed her maid on various things.... By the time she was bathed and dressed, she'd be having nightmares about the traffic jams likely on her way to office. Work and some more work awaited her in office, so the supermom-multi-tasker-career woman would answer her emails on her BB and wave at the urchins while she waited for the lights to go green at the signal. Once at work, she was in another 'zone': conference calls, strategy meetings, pep talks to the team, lend a shoulder to the colleague whose daughter was sick, coordinate for that CSR fund raiser and send a thank you note to the sister-in-law. She did it all with ease; all of it, except for eating.

The last thing on her mind was food. Planning her daughter's lunch box, FiL's lunch and the family's evening meal (her husband had told her that they would manage all meals apart from dinner, and she was oh-so-full of gratitude for his understanding and accommodating nature) had made her so sick that the 'thought of food puts me off'.

Nisha had prepared an Excel sheet and the FiL, husband and daughter had the task of filling it up on a weekly basis. Which they initially did for two-three weeks. Then it was up to Nisha to fill it up keeping in mind everybody's likes and dislikes (her husband did not like ghiya, tori, tendli for dinner; FiL was a Baba Ramdev follower, so he could eat gheeya dudhi every day; and the daughter was usually bored of eating roti sabzi or dal chawal and wanted something more exciting).

'My mom-in-law did it DAILY, babe!' she exclaimed.

'Are you complaining or what?' I asked.

'Just jealous, ya. This whole thing of taking care of these three people ka food fancies gets to me. I have no energy left, seriously, and I don't want to work out, I don't want to enter the kitchen, even if it's just to get a glass of water, I don't want to go to office, I don't want to drive.... Phew! I love my job, trust me. The money, the position, the work —it's all great, no jokes. But now I feel I have no zing left in me. I am doing exciting work with a thakela body, hiding behind long kurtas and black pants and pancake for puffy eyes.'

'You look great to me,' I said. 'It didn't occur to me that you were hiding behind clothes and make-up.'

'Ha ha, I am. I am so hiding. Let me tell you a secret, if you see me without make-up you will freak out, I look nothing short of scary! I can't diet and I can't exercise, so can you still help me?'

'I can't help you even if you *were* ready to exercise and diet. Only you can help yourself, correct na?'

'Yes, meri ma. Tell me what to do. I am trapped, ya.'

'What's your favourite dish?'

'My father-in-law is happy with dudhi in all shapes, sizes and preparations, my daughter freaks out on pav bhaji and my husband on sushi...'

She stopped because I was pointing at her.

'Me? I've been married eleven years now...'

'So it's now illegal to have a favourite dish?'

'Not exactly,' she said smirking. 'But I don't remember what it is. I mean, mere ko sab kuch chalta hai. I am not fussy, I can eat anything they make at home. Okay, my favourite moment is when I go home and nobody asks me what to make or the day when I get food without having to bother what's happening in the kitchen.'

'Okay, so what's your favourite food?' I asked again. Persistence pays — whoever told you that was lying.

'Can I call my mom and ask?'

'You can, but you must know that it's sad that you don't remember. It's precisely this that makes us gain weight — not remembering to eat at the time we like, the food we like and in quantities we like. So you don't need a diet, you need a memory revival of sorts. That you come first; that your food and eating it at the right time and in the right quantities is your responsibility. As an adult and as a working (or non-working) woman, your welfare is your biggest responsibility. So how can you turn your back on yourself under the pretext of work, marriage, children, mom-in-law's untimely death? Your body supports you to carry out all the functions, responsibilities and roles that you have assumed — that of a high-flying career woman, mother, daughter-in-law, bhabi, wife, sister, etc., and what do you do? You behave like an ungrateful bitch who adds insult to all the injuries you inflict upon your body by hiding it!'

'You have no business to talk to me like that!'

'And you have no business hiding your body, Nisha. You buy clothes because you like the colour, the style, the price and not to hide your body. You can't insult your body like this. Be proud, show and decorate your body with clothes and accessories and all that. Take pride in the fact that even after clearly not eating right, not exercising, not sleeping on time, after all this abuse of hiding and stuff your body doesn't turn her back on you. She works for you 24 x 7 and that too unconditionally. Instead of doing meethe shabad and acknowledging that work, you call her fat. She is not fat babe, your body is not fat. She is simply undernourished, overworked and, dare I say, insulted?'

'What do I do, ya? I agree that I am guilty as hell.'

'Nothing big. Just get back to basics. Let's find out what you like eating and you eat that today and let's rework and readjust the way you have been eating from there on.'

So we found out from Nisha's mom that moong dal halwa was her favourite. Yummy, yummy. I helped Nisha decide the right day and timing to eat — so it would be Sunday and after the siesta, around 4 p.m., where she had the time to enjoy her food instead of just 'shoving it down her throat'. Perfect. Post the halwa, it was the Excel sheet, nope not for the family, but for herself. I had asked her to make a trip to her mom's for chai post the halwa and get an Excel sheet for the week ready with her help. Mom was given the responsibility of putting down the recipes for Nisha's favourite sabzis (at least four) and we would use that for her dinners. The other three days were divided between FiL, husband and daughter. Eating their favourite food or whatever was made for them that night. This I think is a great way to eat according to what you like and what the other important family members like.

Women need to start thinking of themselves as being as important as the father-in-law/husband/child/sis-in-law's visiting husband, etc. Only then will they even think of eating right. I mean, will you share somebody else's goodies all your life? How about introducing them to *your* favourite food? And if you don't plan for yourself or think about yourself as important enough to plan or prepare an Excel sheet or a shopping list for, who's to think that for or about you?

Remember what they tell you when you fly: please wear the oxygen mask first before helping your co-passengers or children. So learn to keep yourself well fed first; when you are undernourished and tired there is just no chance that you will do a good job of feeding the rest of the family. Marriage, work pressure, stress or anything else you may think of is not a good enough reason to give up on yourself.

Be kind, be compassionate — to yourself too

Adapt, adjust, accommodate is the philosophy that made Swami Sivananada of Rishikesh, guru to millions around the world. The next line of his philosophy is, 'Be good, do good, be kind, be compassionate'. This second line includes you yourself as well. Not just your family, society, community, country, world, universe. The Advaita philosophy (non-dual) believes that there is no 'other', no 'them' and 'us' — just one nameless, formless reality of absolute bliss (Satchidananda). If you adapt, adjust, accommodate to the external world at the cost of being cruel and harsh to your inner being, the damage, destruction and delusion caused to your inner environment will show in the outer environment too. So want

to keep your husband, children, in-laws happy? Then learn
to keep *yourself* happy first. Or mindless adjustments and
compromises will not just take a toll on your health, hormones
and happiness, but also on theirs.

THE FOUR STRATEGIES

Nutrition strategies	Exercise strategies	Sleep strategies	Relationship strategies
Giving up the food that nourished you to grow from a little girl to a lady is stupid, whatever your marital state.	Giving up on workouts makes you … you know what it makes you — dull and boring.	Weddings and post shaadi may take a toll on quality and quantity of sleep.	Marrying or wanting to marry is not synonymous with being less important than the man.
Preferring to eat at a time different from your husband or in-laws is not a crime. Not listening to your hunger cues is.	It's not about staying thin but about having a life and a body that you are comfy with, so work out.	Return to your regular bed timing as quickly as you can. Work on making your bedroom TV/laptop/BB/iPhone/Playstation and surfing free.	Don't feel guilty if you are not submissive and think differently from your husband. It's totally okay for partners to have different opinions or thought processes, in fact even desirable.
Eat your favourite food at least once every fifteen days, if not once every week.	Increased blood circulation and muscle tone makes you sharp and active in your mind and energetic, attractive in the body.	Waking up tired in the mornings is not 'normal' — the faster you wake up to the fact, the faster you will get fit.	Looking after the home and kitchen is not your exclusive department. Involve and seek your partner's active support. You are living with an adult, not with a little baby or with a lord whom you are now duty-bound to serve.
Supplement your diet with vitamin B because marriages for us are not just physically draining during ceremonies but mentally draining after them.	It also makes your skin glow, increases hair growth and lengthens your nails. So what are you waiting for?		
The lower your calcium intake, the more likely you are to get fat. So work at keeping chai/coffee down and don't forget to take the calcium tablet (calcium citrate — easily absorbed) in the night.			Don't be guilty of not doing/adjusting more than you can handle. Nobody (almost nobody) is going to come to your support when you eventually explode.

Real life diet analysis

Simran Agarwal is a twenty-six-year-old HR consultant. She is a Marwadi girl married to a south Indian.

Within a year of getting married, Simran put on ten kilos, which she believes is due to the changes in her food habits. In a bid to adapt to her husband's lifestyle, she had given up on eating foods she likes and instead ate according to his preferences (so in spite of being a Marwadi, she was eating idlis, dosas, uttapams for breakfast, lunch and dinner!). Whenever her husband travelled, she would eat foods of her choice.

Six years back, she had lost a lot of weight: twenty-five kilos within a year! She had not done the diet or her workout programme under any professional guidance. Her diet had consisted of sprouts, bhel puri, raita, selective vegetables and juices, and she had worked out for three hours every day — gym for an hour and swimming for two hours.

According to Simran, this diet and workout had lead to her having back pain and less stamina.

Her married life was not really working out as she had expected it to, and she had therefore taken up a job to distract herself from this stress, but it was not a job she enjoyed and it only added to her stress, instead of easing it.

She now struggles between work and family life, and along with all this, she is 'trying' very hard to lose weight.

Three-day diet recall

Time	Food/ Drink	Activity Recall	Workout
Day 1			
8.00 a.m.		Woke up, showered, got ready for office	
8.40 a.m.	1 slice brown bread with Amul Lite butter, 1 bowl muesli with cold milk		
10.00 a.m.		Reached office, climbed 3 floors and started work	

11.00 a.m.	1 apple	Took a small break to have my mid-morning snack	
12.30 p.m.		Went for a short meeting (was driven there)	
1.45 p.m.		Returned to office	
2.00 p.m.	2 idlis with sambhar and coconut chutney		
5.30 p.m.		Left office and went to the gym	30-minute walk on treadmill, twenty minutes EFX and 10 minutes cycling
7.15 p.m.		Reached home and took a shower	
8.40 p.m.	2 rotis with channa		
9.00 – 10.30 p.m.		Watched TV	
10.30- 11.00 p.m.		Chatted with husband	
11.00 p.m.		Into bed	
Day 2			
8.00 a.m.		Woke up and got ready for office	
8.40 a.m.	Muesli with cold milk		
10.00 a.m.		Reached office and started work	
11.00 a.m.	1 boiled egg with tossed palak masala, 1 slice brown bread		
1.00 p.m.	2 uttapams with mixed sabzi		
1.30 p.m.		Got back to work	
5.30 p.m.		Left for the day	
6.15 p.m.		Stopped by ATM, picked up groceries	

6.45 p.m.		Went to the gym (Very tired, but had to go and work out! Can't afford to put on any more weight)	1 hour cardio
8.00 p.m.		Got home and took a shower	
8.30 p.m.	Had salad made of potato, beans, carrot, onions with low-fat Caesar dressing and 2 slices of whole wheat bread (husband out of town so I ate food of my choice ☺)		
8.45 p.m.		Washed all dishes	
9.00 – 10.30 p.m.		Watched TV	
10.30 p.m.		Went to sleep	
Day 3 (Holiday)			
8.00 a.m.		Woke up	
8.30 a.m.		Took a shower and got ready for Onam puja	
9.00 a.m.		Did puja at home and sat for breakfast	
9.30 a.m.	2 idlis with tomato chutney		
10.00 a.m.		Went shopping and got home by lunch	
1.30 p.m.	1 bowl of boiled rice with palak dal and masala-tossed yam	Climbed 3 floors to visit friend in building	
2.00 p.m.		Decorated the house for evening puja. Set the table, made my bed, decorated the entrance of the puja room	

5.00 p.m.	2 Marie biscuits	Got ready for guests at home	
6.00 p.m.		Guests arrived. Ran around to get snacks ready and take care of guests	
8.00 p.m.		Guests left. Got dinner ready, cleared the table, and sorted the kitchen	
8.30 p.m.	2 plain dosas with chutney, 1 gulab jamun		
9.00 – 10.30 p.m.		Watched TV, chatted on phone	
10.30 p.m.		Into bed	

Evaluation of the recall

Simran has always been unhappy with her body. At the young age of nineteen, she went on a major crash diet and at the same time started over-exercising because she was desperate to lose weight.

She now hardly eats through the day, as she believes that the food pattern she has adapted to after marriage has contributed to her weight gain. She is tired and exhausted by the end of her day at 5 p.m., but pushes herself to exercise as she believes that this is the least she can do to lose weight.

She really does not care enough about herself and is not doing anything that she likes or enjoys doing — an unsatisfying job, an unhappy marriage — and is unhappy with her body.

Modifications

To begin with, Simran needs to modify her diet and incorporate foods that she likes eating on a daily basis, rather than doing it only when her husband is away.

If Simran starts eating more frequently, and eats foods she likes and as per her genes, she will surely enjoy better stamina and energy levels and will also lose 'fat'. (Absorption and assimilation of nutrients is always better when you eat foods that appeal to your taste buds and foods that you have been traditionally eating. When you eat foods you enjoy, your body is able to secrete the necessary enzymes and digestive juices to digest this food, so you get the best nutrition out of it. If your nutrient requirements are met, you automatically start feeling less stressed out and calmer.)

Also, she needs to take up a more meaningful and satisfying job, something that she can relate to, rather than working at a job just to 'get away' from her unsatisfying married life.

If all this is taken care of, she will enjoy a better state of mind and better energy levels. Instead of compromising on every front, if Simran prioritises herself and does what she likes, she will be more at peace mentally and physically and will be better equipped to sort out her career and married life.

The diet recommended for Simran was as below:

Meal 1 (8.00 a.m., on rising, within 10 mins): Fresh fruit

Meal 2 (8.30 – 9.00 a.m.): Chilla or paratha (something she loves)

Meal 3 (11.00 a.m.): Handful of peanuts/makhana

Meal 4 (1.00 p.m.): Idli/dosa + chutney, sambhar (cannot cook all meals separately for herself, so having this once a day is alright)

Meal 5 (3.00 p.m.): Chaas

Meal 6 (5.00 p.m.): Cheese (she loves it)

Meal 7 (6.30 p.m.): 2 egg whites + 1 whole wheat toast

Meal 8 (8.30 p.m.): Dal/kadhi + sabzi (loves this but hasn't had this ever since she married, except when she goes to her mother's place!)

Simran did find it a little difficult initially to adapt to this eating pattern, because she was not at all used to doing anything for herself and had forgotten what it meant to take care of herself. But as she made an effort, she realised how eating right was making her feel mentally relaxed and that she was not as stressed as she used to be.

She started enjoying her workouts too, and did not have to feel like she was pushing herself to exercise anymore.

She also quit her job as an HR consultant and pursued a career in fashion designing, which she had always wanted to take up. Her husband encouraged her to take this step, and through all this her relationship with her husband also improved.

Simran really does not care much about her weight now, because she has understood the importance of eating right and feeling good mentally and physically. She loves and acknowledges her body for what it is.

4

Pregnancy & Motherhood: The Pain, Trauma & Glory

Pregnancy

In our country, it's like if you are married you *have* to produce a child and yes, quickly. I mean, ya we are very modern so we will give you two years ka window to 'enjoy shaadi', after which you should promptly pop a child out in gratitude for the opportunity to enjoy 'freedom and life' bestowed by your family. If by the fourth year you are not pregnant, you have to start making rounds of all the 'good gynacs' in your neighbourhood/town/city/abroad (how far you go depends on how long you have been 'trying'). Nobody will ask your husband (you know how men are), but everybody will ask you, 'Why are you not having a baby?' and give you dollops of advice on 'Ek baar late then it gets bada mushkil', or lectures on complications with (old) age, and then eventually (unsolicited) sympathy, and then of course the CIDgiri of watching every sentence/look between you and your husband to figure out what's wrong. Why aren't you having a baby? It's already been two/six/ten years!

Getting married is like a licence to have sex and a green signal to pop a baby — it's now legal and binding on you to have a child. Really?

Taku and I were driving into NYC from New Jersey when we came to a crossroad. Taku halted and I started patting his shoulder wildly, shouting, 'Chal, chal, chal, it's a green signal,' pointing to the green traffic light. For the Mumbaikar in me, there was nothing as shameful as not moving (and quickly) when the signal was green, and especially when there was solid traffic. So there we were, in a traffic jam, the intersection was blocked with cars (all single occupancy), and Taku chooses to stop and that too when the signal was green. Ohhh, I was getting impatient and very irritated.

'Arrey, idhar allowed nahi hai,' explained Taku.

'What are you saying? Why they not only drive ulta side, they also stop at green and move on red?'

'Nope, heroine! If the intersection is blocked, you can't move even if the signal is green. You have to wait till it clears. According to the US traffic law, the intersection should always be free.'

Wow! 'Why?'

'Listen, even if we go, we'll get stuck right there and then we'll block traffic for the entire road and from all sides right? I mean we do this in Mumbai all the time, don't we, and then we get frustrated and then everybody on the road is frustrated and nobody moves an inch but everybody is right there, honking, losing tempers, just full on chaos.'

Yes, I had to agree. Similarly, though marriage is a green signal for having a baby, we must first check if our intersection is blocked. Is our fitness levels okay? Work-life okay? Relationship with husband/in-laws okay? Money, home, all okay? All clear? Then move ahead and have your baby. If not, allow the blocks in the different areas of your life to clear. Or else be prepared for a frustrating and chaotic experience.

Real life example
'I don't know why I'm telling you this ... it's not even related to our topic, but...'

Go ahead, I said.

'Five days ago I was at one of the birthday parties that my son was invited to and they gave us this dumb puzzle that we had to solve. And I just couldn't work it out. I just couldn't! I was staring at this dumb thing and I couldn't work it out!' Eyes welling up now. 'I don't know who this is inside of me and what I have become in the last three years!'

Aayah! I said to myself. Thoroughly ashamed, I worked at maintaining the practiced calm on my face. Prabha was talking again. 'I am from LSE and what am I doing now? Raising two children: a three-year-old boy and a one-year-old daughter. Going with one for a birthday party, taking the other to the park, tired, exhausted, sleepless and fat! You know, this is not how I used to be just four years ago. That's not so LONG ago, right?' I shook my head, no that's not long ago. 'I was gymming regularly, running thirty minutes on the treadmill, fitting into whatever I wanted and solving puzzles, crosswords, sudoko like this,' she snapped her fingers, 'this fast. And now I look at the treadmill at home and I feel nauseous and guilty as hell. I stare at a dumb birthday party puzzle and I can't work it out. I feel like an old, dull hag ...' tears finally on the high cheekbones. 'You know what I wanted? Two children before thirty! I just wanted to finish it off.

Because post-thirty it's supposed to be tough and all that. Wah! What an achievement! I am such a loser.

'You know I don't get enough time with my husband, even he is like why are you like this all the time? The worst thing is there is nothing I can complain about! My husband is sweet and understanding and makes a great father. He plays with them every night after he is back from work and after I put them to sleep, he is like — okay, let's spend some time together. He just wants me to sit and watch some TV with him. So you know, I am forcing myself to keep my eyes open and watch whatever he is watching, and sometimes I notice that he has dozed off. Sirf wo abhi uthke sab band karo, light, TV and stuff drains me out. Here I am trying to stay up to spend time together, he has dozed off and I get to switch off the lights and put the remote back in its place.

'My mother-in-law is also very sweet. Sometimes I feel guilty that I am just using her. I go out for lunch at times, once or twice a month, and she readily takes care of the kids. Even if I get late, she won't say a word. Of course I have maids and all that, but you know how it is, kitne bhi maids ho, when it is kids, you've got to be on your toes man, 24 x 7. Now my husband is saying let's go away for this long weekend, just somewhere close to Delhi, Gurgaon types, I would so love to go but I just can't. Where will I go with two kids? Then I have to take the maids and he doesn't want to go with the maids. But without the maids it'll be a nightmare.

'When I'm at home, all that I feel like doing is sleeping. Post lunch I want to sleep, in the morning after my husband leaves and Rudra goes to school, I want to sleep, in the night while watching TV during our "me time" I want to sleep. I JUST want to sleep. I don't understand what is happening! I am just not the person I used to be. I love my kids, simply adore them but after them my life is phut! Gone by ... going by ... and I don't know what I am doing. Sleeping?'

Are you? I asked.

'No, no, not in the day. I have too many things to do, look after my daughter, then my son comes home, so feed him lunch and then in the evening I go out with them to the park or something. I like doing activities with them or else they get so cranky sitting at home. As it is I feel like I'm a terrible mother so I want to spend time with them, do things with them, play and all ... so that ... okay, I don't believe I'm telling you this, but I'm very insecure! I feel if I don't do all these things, they won't love me, they will forget me.'

'Oh come on ... which child will forget ...'

'You don't know Rujuta. Sometimes when I come back from one of my lunches — I barely go once in two weeks — but after I'm back my daughter won't come to me. She prefers being with the maid. I can't explain how it makes me feel. It's terrible, it's like being punished for going out for lunch, for spending time without her, for leaving her alone. My husband thinks I am over-reacting and tells me babies are moody so I shouldn't make a big deal about it. But it's a big deal for me. VERY big. I have quit everything for them and then this is what I get in return. I feel like a failure on all fronts. I wish I could come back home happy and have the kids running to me instead of being at home and doing everything for them.

'Do I sound like a bitch? I mean I have everything, a good husband, a supportive family, a good education, two lovely children and this is how I feel … I am really a …'

'Misinformed person,' I offered.

'Is that an euphemism for ungrateful?'

'No, it's the apt word for your state. I know my English, ya.'

Big smile from Prabha now, and shoulders finally moving away from the ears to a more relaxed state (thank god). Yes, the word is misinformed. A highly-educated, smart girl with no understanding of what her body has gone through and misinformed about what she needs to do to set things right.

Eating right, working out, sleeping on time and allowing for good rest and recovery — if Prabha had done all this before getting pregnant the first time, and especially before the second time, then she wouldn't be as drained out, dazed and guilty as she is feeling. To feel upbeat and yummy post kids, it's crucial to plan for this physically and emotionally draining phase in advance, way in advance. Prabha was chasing the figure 'thirty'. 'They say' it's difficult post thirty. It's difficult at any stage and at any age, and lack of physical fitness only compounds the difficulty. It's not age which makes pregnancy easy or difficult. **A fit and well-nourished body is what makes pregnancy easy, and it is really not dependent on age.** Come on, we come from India, nobody knows this better than us. A lot of young women, sometimes as young as fifteen and as 'old' as twenty-three, who are nutritionally deprived have tough pregnancies and complicated deliveries, including infections and blood loss; some of them even die in childbirth. So it's not age; if anything, the ease comes with nourishment and fitness.

The frozen egg

'So when are you freezing your eggs?' 'What??' Yeh sunne ke pehle asman phat kyun nahi gaya, dharti tut kyun nahi gaya and whatever. 'When are you freezing your eggs?' Neeraja repeated her question as I stared blankly at her. 'You should do it soon, you know. Before thirty you have the best eggs. To conceive you need the best eggs and the best sperm, you know? You are already thirty-two!! Now by the time you get married and you have children it will get really late, you know.' 'What are you talking about babe?' I said (in my mind). Neeraja's monologue continued: 'My sister just celebrated thirty-five years ka birthday, she is not married yet and we are looking for a boy for her but we have frozen her eggs.' Wow! I could picture the sister getting married and the husband getting frozen eggs in dowry. 'You should do that too — use technology, use it to freeze your eggs.'

Neeraja was the president of a women's club and I had been invited as a guest speaker for one of their functions. Neeraja had sung my praises and said the club had had to wait over six months and cough up my fees to get me, blah blah. Now, in the evening, as she dropped me home in her chauffer-driven Merc, LV on her arm, Choos on her feet and carats all over, she was going bananas over my 'old age', 'unmarried' and 'childless' status, and my 'dark future'. So I was receiving unsolicited sympathy and advice about what to do to have children, and I was thinking maybe I should have a clause: 'If the organisers of the workshop say idiotic things to me then they need to pay a penalty, four or five times my fees, for not knowing when to shut up!' No, I still haven't added the clause, but maybe I really should.

It's like this. We may call you for a talk, lend you an ear and probably even look up to you and applaud your 'achievements', but at the end of it, 'there is truly no achievement bigger than becoming a mother'. Should I have told her that motherhood is enjoyed most when it's 'chosen' and not when it's 'frozen' or mindlessly complied to or chased before reaching some kind of imaginary deadline? Child-bearing, rearing, tending is rewarding when it comes out of choice, not out of a sense of 'achievement'.

Preparing for pregnancy

Pregnancy drains a woman's body of all, okay, *most* of its resources. I mean, how many of us plan to equip our body a year in advance before getting pregnant? How many of us plan for the US visa a year (okay, months) in advance, get our paperwork in place and find the right agent? And how many of us know how to dress up our résumé to land that dream job? How many of us plan for dinners and get the house in order, cleaned, stocked and equipped to deal with guests? Does anybody need an education or book to learn how to plan in advance for what we'll wear at a cousin's wedding? Nah. We don't need that. We are awesome planners and we can plan backwards with perfection. But somehow it never strikes us that if the house needs to be cleaned, stocked and equipped to deal with a guest, the body might need to be cleaned of disease and discomfort, stocked with nutrients and equipped with the right attitude to welcome this 'new growth' or baby. A baby, after all, is a nine-month guest in a woman's body. And like a well-meaning guest, it can prove to be a parasite if the body doesn't have the infrastructure to allow its optimum growth. Nature has its own laws and it has decided that the baby gets precedence over the mother. So if the woman's body is not receiving enough dietary nutrients, the foetus will get its due from the body's reserve.

Folic acid and calcium supplements

Sorry to tell you this, but the symbolic 'strengthening' of the body with folic acid and calcium supplements is just as effective as appointing a woman for the post of president of India. Has the fate of our women changed? Does having Pratibha Patil as the president mean fewer female infanticides, no glass ceiling, insurance cover for your parents and drastic reduction in dowry deaths? No. But is it a symbol of how far Indian women have come? Yes, she gets to be the president of this country. And you still get to do the dishes. Good deal?

Symbolism is just that — symbolic. For real change to happen, it takes time and planning. So take the supplements your gynaecologist has prescribed, but eat serious, nutritious food even before you stop using the condom/pill. **When the body gets its due of nutrient-rich carbs, protein and fat (I mean unprocessed, tazaa ghar ka khana), then the folic acid and calcium supplements work like a miracle.** Without the nutrients, they remain just symbolic. If you are popping pills, make it meaningful.

Make a woman president meaningful by doing solid and genuine work on the ground. Symbolism unsupported by real change and work is hypocrisy.

Oral health

How soon should you start the clean-up act? Well, to begin with, you shouldn't be dirtying your body with junk food, unhealthy bedtimes and inactivity in any case. But if you have been doing all this, it's never too early or late to start. So, of course, start by cleaning up your digestive system and start from the very beginning. Go to a dentist and get all those things done that you've been putting off. There is research that points towards the fact that better teeth and chewing = fewer urinary tract and vaginal infections. Something that almost every mother/pregnant woman will confess to having, to a lesser or greater degree. Better chewing and stronger gums also mean less bloating and better moods, so better chances of fertility. Not just that, but better chewing and breaking down of food in your stomach will mean better digestion and optimum response of hormones like insulin. Optimum insulin response is crucial for your cells to receive the nutrients from the food you consume. Start at least twelve months prior to stopping your condom/pill. That way, after cleaning your teeth, gums, cavities, you have the time to go for at least one follow-up session with your dentist to ensure that your oral health is stable. Oral health is one of the most overlooked aspects of 'getting pregnant' and having a 'normal delivery'.

Right nutrition

Both parents need to be fit, but since this is a book for women, I am going to spare you gyaan about men, their fitness, density and the speed of sperms, and focus on ovaries, hormones and nutrition for women. The ovaries can maintain perfect hormonal harmony if you are willing to eat right. Read that again — if you are willing to *eat right*; not if you *lose weight*. Women who are 'trying', are told by their gyny that everything is alright, you just need to 'lose weight'. Now when your doctor is saying lose weight, what it essentially means is 'get fitter', so learn to read between the lines. If you fall sick before your next appointment with your doctor and lose weight as a consequence (weight loss follows illness/sickness/surgery, etc.), it doesn't improve your chances of getting pregnant; if anything, it hampers it. And please, our doctors are too busy and have to meet their next client immediately, so they won't have the time to explain all this to you. So use common sense and what can be understood by lagaoing a little dimaag shouldn't be understood at the cost of chabaoing the doctor's brain and by eating into their 'precious' time.

Sorry, no offence, doctors — perhaps they don't realise that their words have such a profound effect on the lives of their patients. Women run frantically from one diet fad to another, losing weight unhealthily and at the cost of depleting and destroying their nutritional status. Poor eating habits or fads (today only dudhi, tomorrow only dal; fibre drink before meals; tea/coffee to kill appetite, etc.) further reduce chances of getting pregnant, and even if you do get pregnant, it almost ensures that there is an associated unhealthy weight gain during pregnancy, making the period of pregnancy (a beautiful period in a woman's life and also a very special time for everybody around her) difficult and tiring, and complicating the process of delivery.

The focus should instead stay on developing a nutritionally richer status. So cut back on tea/coffee, stop smoking and drinking (yeah, even wine), start eating according to the four principles (detailed in Introduction) and Nutrition Strategies (Chapter 7) and work on achieving regular meal timings and on eating fresh, unprocessed, in-season food grown with minimum or zero pesticides and chemicals. Eating right and at the right time ensures a good response from all the hormones of your body, specifically your insulin, which becomes so sharp and alert with the nourishment that it ensures that every cell in your body is well nourished.

Another big reason to eat right is so your mood remains happy and stable. Fluctuating blood sugars (the consequence of a fasting-and-feasting pattern) will leave you depressed and low. I mean, you are hardly going to feel up to sex. Steady, stable blood sugars keep you happy, energetic and in the mood for sex. Now if you are going to be making babies, you might as well enjoy the whole process from the beginning to the end, and the middle, of course. When a baby is conceived out of love, it's much more fun and meaningful than a baby conceived out of 'I have to have sex today — it's my date'. Then you are just rocking and not enjoying the party.

Pointers for what to eat during pregnancy

1. Eat a fruit along with a handful of dry fruits within ten minutes of waking up.
2. Have a homemade nutritious breakfast one hour after the fruit. Avoid bread, biscuits, pickles and sauces at this time.
3. Have lunch by between 11 a.m. to max 1 p.m. Don't delay this meal.
4. Eat a variety of cereals (like whole wheat, jowar, bajra, rice, nachni, rajgira, etc.) for lunch along with fresh veggies and a dal.
5. Have curd or chaas post lunch after a two-hour gap. Avoid adding salt and sugar, but feel free to add fresh black pepper or jeera.
6. Preferably cut down on chai/coffee to not more than one cup a day (also made at home).
7. Include cheese, paneer, peanut butter, white butter (homemade) for a snack or early dinner by 6-7 p.m. This meal could be similar to lunch, but with one of the above mentioned options.
8. Eat seasonal sabzi or steamed veggies with a small bowl of khichdi or kadhi by 9 p.m.
9. Stay active during the day and walk around as much as possible. Avoid sitting in one place for a long time.

> 10. Drink plenty of water and stay well hydrated throughout the pregnancy and post-delivery stage.
> 11. Be regular with your vitamin and mineral supplements.

Work out

Eating right, making sure there's wholesome food on your plate and regularising meal timings is one aspect of keeping physically fit. Now every woman wants a 'normal' delivery and we all want to look like million bucks, and if possible younger and skinnier post pregnancy, but for that you need another aspect of keeping fit in place — EXERCISE. To feel up to exercise (and sex), the body has to be well nourished. Without good food and disciplined meal timings, it's impossible to nourish the system, and without the required 'energy' to work out and recover, you will feel down and make mindless excuses to avoid or skip exercise: I'll start from this Monday/arrey I first need to buy better tights/not today because I don't feel like washing my hair/I am bored, ya, etc. If you genuinely want to exercise but haven't started, it's just poor nutritional status. No, it's not laziness, or lack of discipline.

What's 'trying to get pregnant' got to do with workouts? Well, everything. For starters, a lack of blood circulation makes conception difficult. A well worked out body has better muscle and bone density, which has an anti-ageing effect so you now have a biologically younger body whatever your chronological age may be. Regular workouts increase your pain threshold, so you just walked a step closer to a 'normal' delivery, and yes, they also make your back, pelvis, legs stronger, so that's a few more steps closer to a 'normal' delivery and staying fit during and post pregnancy. What else? Well you won't have back pain, leg pain, swollen feet during and post pregnancy because of the stronger and better capillary and nerve network in the body. The uterus will be stronger and better nourished, so no sagging post pregnancy, and ya, the boobs won't sag either.

What kind of a workout should you do? Well, weight-training, yoga asanas, Pilates, cycling, running, everything works — but it's got to be more than just walking. Like I said earlier, it's not about 'weight loss', it's about getting fitter and improving chances of getting pregnant, staying pregnant and delivering normally.

Fitness has four major components: flexibility, strength, cardio-respiratory fitness and body fat percentage. (See Exercise Strategies in Chapter 7) You've got to improve and build better flexibility, strength, cardio-respiratory fitness and lean body weight (stronger muscles + denser bones). Only then will body fat levels drop, and yes, body weight will drop too. And oh yes, with regular workouts, you also lose less blood during delivery and your menstrual cycle will stay regular prior to and post pregnancy. Have I managed to sell you exercise? Ah! One more — stronger and healthier eggs, foetus and a baby with less chance of turning into an obese adult. The list really is endless.

Diet for life

When you're 'trying', the other thing doctors will tell you is, 'Don't go on a diet now; you will need to get off your diet when you're pregnant.' Now to begin with, **a 'diet' is something that you should be able to stay with for your life**; it's not something that you drop like a hot potato when you get pregnant. So, ensure that the 'diet' you are on makes it easier for you to get pregnant, to stay pregnant (comfortably) and to deliver normally. It has to have all the major nutrients, carbs, proteins, fat and all the essential vitamins and minerals and, yes, water too. Don't expect your doctor to find out if you are on a fad diet or on a 'realistic change in lifestyle, sleeping on time, eating on time, eating right, working out regularly, staying fit' diet. You need to lagao your dimaag. If you are eating sensibly according to the four principles (see Introduction) and Nutrition Strategies (Chapter 7), it's a 'diet' you must stay on during pregnancy (after pregnancy and for the rest of your life). You can't blame your doctor for saying get off the 'diet' when you're pregnant. Diet has become synonymous with starvation. And if you are going to be starving during your pregnancy, you are going to create trouble for yourself for all nine months yes, but also for your doctor on the delivery table.

How essential fatty acids help

We all know by this time that during our periods we lose the all-important calcium through our menstrual blood. Calcium loss is the main reason for cramps, dullness and bloating during PMS and the menstrual cycle. Now, during pregnancy, hold your breath, you lose *four times* the amount of calcium that you would have lost had you gotten your periods in those nine months. So in those nine months, your bones and body can age up to four years or more, depending on how fit, nourished and sensible you have been before getting pregnant. And that's just one of the reasons why this jazz of planning in advance is crucial. And so is working out, eating right and sleeping on time — it's all to build those calcium banks, have a healthy foetus and make it easier for yourself to get back in shape post pregnancy.

Another reason to be on a sensible diet (not starvation) before and during pregnancy is essential fatty acids. The most common (and disastrous) implication of the word 'diet' is reduction in calories best achieved by reducing dietary fat (all in the hope of losing body fat — how did we go SO wrong). A blanket ban on fats (just like the blanket ban doctors put on 'diet') is stupid, to say the very least. Essential fats that you get from sources like nuts, including peanuts, groundnut oil, til oil, homemade ghee, cheese, homemade butter, milk, paneer, fish, flaxseeds, coconut, olives, etc. improve your and your baby's immune system (we don't want them falling ill, right?) and sharpens their brains (we want them to do well in school and life, right?). Fats help the baby grow, and help their brain cells as well. The next time you see your little child displaying her ability to solve a puzzle/memorise verses/analyse — touch your butt gently and say a silent thank you. It's thanks to your fat cells that her brain is that smart, alert and sharp. So keep the fats in your diet, eat the ghee, don't switch to baked and low-fat products and don't forget to sleep well.

Eating for two

There is only one person while you're connected through that umbilical cord, so don't eat that ice cream and say 'your baby needs it', or that chocolate cake because 'your baby wants it'. It's you. And more than you, it's your nutrient deficiencies. If you'd eaten sensibly and what you require all through your life, you'll never feel the need to eat for two when you're pregnant. Stay in touch with your body now, and with how much you eat, and what you need. You have no access to the baby's stomach. The foetus can, in fact, make do with the reserves available. If your appetite has increased, feel free to eat more, but know that it's because your body needs it, not the baby. Oh, and those cravings for pickle and chocolate just mean that there are nutritional deficiencies or you're watching too many Hindi movies.

Assume the responsibility

A major problem that I have seen with women is that they shirk responsibility at the time of delivery. Almost every pregnant woman tells her gyny — 'Doctor mujhe kuch bhi karke NORMAL delivery chahiye.' Hello! Hello!! Wake up! Doing 'kuch bhi' is *your* responsibility, not your doctor's. If you have poor fitness levels, nutrient deficiencies, low pain tolerance, tight hamstrings, a stiff pelvic area and all that, what's the doctor going to do? You've got to address these issues even before thinking of getting pregnant and take full responsibility to ensure a normal delivery. Remember it's your vagina and your womb, your foetus and your uterus — YOU have got to keep them healthy and strong (not your doctor, for heaven's sake).

Women in cities like Mumbai often complain that they had to go through Caesarean while their cousin in some small town went through normal delivery. It's not that all doctors here are keen on making more money. They mostly just have women patients that are fatter, have poorer fitness levels, and who have less access to fresh local food as compared to women in villages or smaller towns. And please, if you are good with maths, think about this — less money with a normal delivery, but also less time, less effort (ya, you also have to push, not your doctor), less number of nights you occupy their bed, so isn't that called a fast 'turnover', which means that I can accommodate more patients in the same number of days, with less effort, less time and happier patients: as a gyny, what would I choose? Am I promoting gynys and dentists? Do I have gyny and dentist friends? Yes. Am I getting paid for it? No ya. What I am really trying to do (and hopefully with some degree of success) is to tell you that a normal delivery is very much a possibility if you work at it, but you need to work at it a year in advance (prior to conception), and not *after* you get pregnant.

Jhadu-katka methods

Here's another thing women do which so totally beats common sense. In the ninth month most women get impatient and all they want to do is deliver asap, and yes, 'normally'. So they hear all these stories like 'want to deliver fast and normal just do some jhadu-katka in the house'. So the tigresses emerge from their den with a broom and bucket all set to sweep, swab and 'deliver'. They totally overlook the fact that they may not have done this their entire lives, or that they have been put on bed rest or that they have never even been to a gym or worked out before this — so now just a week or two before delivery, why all the cleaning, lifting, pulling, pushing? Though we live in a world of Instant coffee and noodles, 'normalcy' during pregnancy, while delivering and post pregnancy, comes from planning and effort in the right direction, and it's much more than 'just do jhadu in the last week'. Women invariably pull or strain some body part (especially around the weight bearing joints — hip, lower back, knee, ankle) during this overzealous activity when the last thing that you should be risking is an injury. A protruding stomach is challenging enough for the back, why are you then adding uneven forces on the spine with jhadu-katka?

Work out and improve circulation by all means, but in a sensible manner. It's important to stay fit during pregnancy, but it's also equally important to not introduce exercise (especially without expert supervision) randomly on getting the 'good news'. So really, the best option is get fit before conceiving and then stay fit through out, all those nine months and later through life.

Real life example

My friend Bhavana had been working out (weight-training in the gym for more than five years, running the Mumbai half-marathon for two years, and yoga over a year) regularly, ate totally right, enjoyed good levels of fitness and shared a warm, loving relationship with her husband, Mahesh. Married for almost ten years, they were bogged down with questions and requests for 'good news'. It's not that they wanted to keep the good news away, but it wasn't coming in the way of their marriage and life either. Bhavz was over the moon with the news of her pregnancy, and so were all of us. She kept up with regular workouts and thought that prenatal classes were too lame for her fitness levels. And she then delivered normally (not once did she or her doctor think she wouldn't). Her baby is now only a month old and Bhavz is the coolest and most energetic mother I have ever seen. Waking up to feed her baby, bathing, playing, carrying, lifting, etc. look like such effortless physical tasks, that I often tell her that she is an advertisement for getting pregnant. Mahesh, on his part, makes a great dad and contributes much more than men usually do, and now feels very strongly that when and whether to get pregnant at all has to be entirely the woman's decision. He recently confessed that he now feels that men can do so little, especially in the initial phases of a baby's life — carrying them in a womb, labour, recovering from delivery and then feeding, nursing the baby, etc. that men should have no say in this matter. Bhavz was only thirty-six years old when she delivered, but it's her workouts, disciplined lifestyle and a loving partner that made her pregnancy, delivery and post-pregnancy seem like a cakewalk.

Netala

At my yoga ashram in Netala, a small Himalayan village near Uttarkashi, women start their day very early and work all year round. They do hard-core physical work, day in and day out. During one of my yoga courses, there was a woman staying near-by who was pregnant almost full term with her first baby. I was amazed at how she never fussed that she was pregnant, instead carrying on with her life as if nothing had happened. Where I come from, women won't bend, carry, lift, climb, exercise, walk … in fact, a lot of them take complete bed rest. One day, as I walked into a yoga session at 4.15 p.m., we noticed that all the women had come home very early. We heard that the pregnant woman had started her labour pains. By the time we'd finished our session at 6.30 p.m., she'd already had her baby and was feeling good enough to lie on the charpoy outside the room where she'd delivered!

I wondered why back home (read cities), pregnancy is treated like a disease. Why just pregnancy, menopause and your period every month are treated like diseases, instead of what they are — a natural part of a woman's life.

After the baby

Motherhood: perhaps, perhaps not the bravest thing a woman can do in her lifetime is give birth to her baby. For this she uses her strongest muscle, the uterus, capable of bearing the load of a full-grown baby in the nine months of pregnancy. Of course, we all love our 3-D scans and the sight of the baby, but do we remember to thank the uterus or pause for a second to acknowledge the work its doing for us. Had it not been for the fact that it moves down a bit after pregnancy, we would have almost let it perish without notice. But we, like strict school teachers, notice that it's moved and complain, Oh! It's sagging. Will my stomach ever look flat again? Of course it will. More on that later, for now know that even when it does, we don't thank it for moving back or encourage it with a gesture of kindness or appreciation, we just let it go back to a zindagi of anonymity.

Strength and resilience are two things nature armed you (the uterus is both strong and resilient) with. To be brave is the intrinsic nature of women. Social conditioning has made us believe otherwise, but when you or your sister or friend or any woman you are really close to delivers a baby, it's like Mother Nature holding a mirror up to you: see, bravery comes easy to you, why not use it more often in your life.

Hirkani

Hirkani was a working mother (now, of course, this term should be banned) and she sold milk in Raigad, Shivaji Maharaj's capital and a fort that he was proud of. Strong and resilient, this was one fort that was practically impossible for the enemy to attack or escape from. The gates of this massive fort would close everyday by 7 p.m., after which nobody could leave or enter this well-guarded and brilliantly built fort on top of a hill. It was an engineering marvel. Now it's an archaeological marvel, and like most heritage sites in our country, in a state of disrepair. Maharashtra has more than one political party claiming to champion the cause of the Marathi manoos; our forts and other sites of 'Marathi culture' are, however, orphaned. The awesomely built courtroom and market of the Raigad fort is frequented by unruly men who go up there for 'programme' — Marathi slang for getting drunk. They leave the bottles behind, along with plastic wrappers of chakna and chips, but that's another story.

Here's the real story. So back then there weren't any ropeways and Hirkani lived in one of the villages at the foothills. She would walk up the hill, carrying a load of pots of milk over her head, and then sell the milk in the market of Raigad. One day Hirkani had a particularly long day at trading her milk. She rushed back to make it to the gates before they closed, under all circumstances she had to reach home. Time however doesn't wait for anybody, not even for a mother when all that she wants to do is to be with her baby, hold the little baby by her breast and feed her. So the gates were already locked and no amount of pleading, begging with the guards would help. Shivaji Maharaj's laws were strict and it was unthinkable to break them. Hirkani however felt that laws or rules which keep a mother away from her baby need to be bypassed, even if it meant getting the ruler of her state angry.

The closed gates broke her heart but not her spirit. She made her way back to the market and surveyed the entire fort to look for an opening. There was one, a really treacherous vertical drop. Motherhood empowers women to overcome the biggest hurdles, both mentally and physically. Throwing caution to the wind, the brave mother made her way down to her village and back to her baby. Next morning she was back to selling milk in the fort, badly bruised but unbroken in her spirit.

When the guards saw Hirkani entering the fort in the morning, they were dumbstruck; it was impossible for the mightiest of warriors to leave the fort after the gates were closed, let alone a young fragile woman. When they reported the case to Shivaji, he was so touched by Hirkani's bravery and unrelenting spirit that he named the drop as Hirkanicha kada or Hirkani's drop (you can see it even today and only marvel at how anyone could have even thought of climbing down there — you won't even want to rapple down, it's that dead-straight a drop). He of course didn't just stop at naming the drop (again very unlike the political parties who claim to be led and inspired by him) after her, he actually relaxed and reviewed his rules and saw Hirkani's point totally — any law which troubles the people it is meant to protect needs to be reviewed and, if necessary, revoked.

Real life example: A study in unfeasibility

'Almost everything post a baby becomes like a feasibility study,' philosophised Shweta, mother of a nine-month-old. 'You know, I don't remember what my life was like before Nivaan. It's madness now, but I can't imagine life without him either. Everything revolves around his food time, potty, nap — it's like I don't exist. I don't remember the last time I went to a parlour to wax; even my eyebrows are just growing, and manicure-pedicure toh, I think I did it in my last janam or something. And I am still wearing some of those pregnancy clothes. Yeh dekh,' she said as she stood up and pulled the elastic of her pants.

'Wow! It can fit three of you.'

'I know, it's sick. I want to get back into some real clothes now. For heaven's sake, everything's like sadaoing in my wardrobe. I tried these jeans the other day. I could wear them till I was almost five months pregnant, no jokes, but they are not going up beyond my knees. Can you beat that? It's taken me nine months to try them and then they don't go above my knees! I was like I need a diet or I should just get pregnant again, because I can't afford to look like a balloon anymore. But getting pregnant is not happening because I so hate my body now that I have lost all interest in sex. I dread to look at myself, so imagine what Deepak must be feeling! And kabhi agar on some random occasion I do finally feel like it, I have to do another study on how much time I have till Nivaan wants his next feed/potty/nap, etc. So I am like doing this feasibility study all the time. Is it feasible to have sex/eat lunch/go to the parlour/talk on the phone/go for a movie without hampering his schedule? The answer is usually NO! So I am changing the name to unfeasible study!!'

'Oh!! So sorry ya...'

'Arrey no, no don't get me wrong, I love him to death and poor thing is just dependent on me for everything ya, from poo to food to sleep to nappy to play, so I have to be there for him. I can't be selfish and just do what I want.'

'What *do* you want?'

'Haan?'

'What do you want?'

'No nothing, thanks. Anyway, I have been eating too much and drinking too much tea.'

'Arrey no, you were saying na, that Nivaan depends on you for everything so you can't just do what you want and be selfish.'

'Oh, that. Stuff like working out and going for a movie or a massage or at least waxing. But I can't do it because I want to do my best for him. I don't want to be selfish. But I want to get thin also, ya. I am like mother dairy you know, just feeding, and Deepak cracks this terrible one on me: "Why do cows have long faces? So would you if somebody would only pull your breasts and not have sex!" So I feel like I am this long-faced cow, no sex and no interest in life and wearing maternity clothes abhi tak and generally looking like a mother. Okay, let me tell you, I don't want to look like a mother, I just want to be the most perfect, the most ideal mother to Nivaan.'

'You are already perfect and ideal, ya.'

'Shut up.'

'I really mean it. You are not doing anything for yourself and you've made your life revolve around your baby; doesn't that just automatically make you an ideal mother?'

This is a (really unnecessary) battle that mothers have to fight. This whole thing about being an 'ideal mother', and before that, 'an ideal wife'. It's like our life is wasted if we don't become these things. Most women with time will eventually resign themselves to the fact that they can't, or that it's beyond them, to be the 'ideal wife', but they will die before giving up on trying to be an 'ideal mother'. And hello, what is an ideal mother? The one who puts her child above everything else and mostly over herself? This attitude is supposed to give us all the fulfilment and happiness in life; women however often don't feel anywhere close to happy. Taking care of our home, husband, children (again, not really in this order), ensuring that they get the best to eat, the time to relax, an environment to achieve their fullest potential, giving them garam rotis (made in the 'healthiest' oils), medicines, tonics, clean clothes, undies, etc. is the biggest contribution that we can make in our lifetime, and is rewarding, satisfying and enriching — or at least that's what we are conditioned to believe.

Let's assume it really is; even then, to provide for them in such a manner will require a really strong, responsible and enthusiastic woman. A woman who has forgotten to look after herself and, more specifically, her basic needs — food, sex and sleep — can never expect to be strong, responsible and enthusiastic. She is (you got that right) guilty, frustrated, tired and, above all, fat. **Frankly speaking, a little baby who is dependent on you for poo to food and everything in between shouldn't be**

burdened with the complex task of making you feel happy or complete as well.

Security, happiness and completeness have nothing to do with husband, marriage, children or their grades or whatever. It lies (cliché, cliché) within. To reach deep within your real being, you will first need to get your body in shape, nourish it with food, love, and the often overlooked and underappreciated aspect, peaceful sleep.

So though Shweta had made all the sacrifices necessary to be an 'ideal mother', she didn't feel like one. Ideal mothers are all very happy, she told me. 'You know, in ads, these skinny women they show as mothers are always grinning ear to ear whether they are cleaning their baby's chubby butts with wipes or making baby food. I am like — huh, I never feel like that. I love Nivaan to death, but every time I sit down to eat is when he does potty, and I know I have to clean it, you know, but I am like, why now?? I can't tell you how it feels. Am I sounding like an idiot?'

'No ya, you sound perfectly NORMAL. Every mother on earth who loves her child to death wishes that the baby didn't do potty or susu while she was eating or, after the baby grows up, that he/she doesn't ask important questions or talk to her when she is in the bathroom.'

'Really? You think so?'

'I am ready to bet my life on it, so stop feeling guilty. You probably just need a little more help on the home front. That's the one thing mothers need, more help from the rest of the family. Does Deepak help (or does he just crack jokes)?'

'Ya, he does, but you know Nivaan wants only me. And anyway men don't have that maternal instinct also, na.'

'Get off it ya. First of all there is no proven "maternal instinct" out there.'

'Kya bolti hai yaar? Sachhi?'

'There is only the instinct to have sex, which of course is second only to the instinct to survive. So it's like this: if I am surviving I might as well have sex.'

'Kya bolti hai? Rubbish!'

Sex

Weight loss without an improvement in the nutritional status and fitness levels is like a fake orgasm. You look like you have achieved it or 'arrived', but deep within you feel cheated, hollow, shunned and depressed. A real orgasm is achieved by expressing yourself freely and fearlessly, it's an extension of the love you share with your body and your partner, it transcends beyond the physical, biochemical reactions. It's something which calms you and uplifts you at the same time; it affects and is affected by much more than the mere physical relationship. Having sex because it's a particular day or date of your menstrual cycle makes sex tiresome, boring, mechanical and 'end-result' driven. It's no longer about enjoying the process or journey, it's all about what we get in the end. This mostly leaves both partners in such a bad frame physically, mentally and emotionally, that even when pregnancy follows it feels like 'target achieved' or 'burden off my shoulders' than really a celebration of spontaneous, fearless lovemaking. To get back to a healthy sex life post pregnancy, it's important to have one before getting pregnant. Without a return to a healthy and loving physical relationship with your partner, the 'yummy mummy' tag will be a drain.

Survival, sex, food and sleep

'Seriously, basic human instincts (those common to all humans irrespective of gender, culture, geography, religion, time, etc.) are only four: survival, sex, food and sleep. Often also called as the four primitive fountains of life. There are still tribes untouched by "civilisation" that look down upon child-bearing or mothering so this whole maternal instinct is plain jazz or at best as true as "paternal instinct". A by-product of our instinct to have sex is to have off-spring or children. Biologically, the mother or the female gets pregnant, delivers and feeds; males lack the required equipment. But our biology, babe, should be our virtue/advantage, na, not something that ties us down to specific roles or makes us fat! We are constantly made to feel that we don't do enough as mothers; almost every mother that I know feels far from ideal. And this is one thing which saddens me the most, seriously. Have you been to a wildlife sanctuary?'

'I told you na, I haven't even been to a parlour.'

'Ya, okay. Seen pictures of elephants? Have you seen that the baby elephant is often surrounded by a lot of adult elephants — you can't make out which one is the mother. The entire herd is taking part in bringing up, protecting and providing for the baby.'

'Arrey I am feeling fucked now. I even *look* like an elephant, so where is my team?'

'Two things. One, if you called yourself an elephant in a bad way, then it's not done. Elephants are beautiful and the most intelligent animals on earth, so if it was meant as a compliment, I am okay, but...'

'Okay sorry meri ma.'

'Okay, two. Maybe your team is around and you are not letting them take part in the process because you are carrying some burden of "maternal instinct" or feel insecure that you don't do enough for your child. Do you know what the most priceless thing for a little baby or for any child is? A healthy, happy and a self-assured mother. Somebody who knows that by investing an hour in the gym she actually provides and ensures that the child will have a happy childhood with a spirited mother who can bend forwards, backwards, run, jump and not have swollen feet, weak knees and a bad back. A mother who eats intelligently, enjoying and relishing the flavour, taste and aroma of food, so that her hormones are regulated and she never feels unduly agitated, angry or low. A mother who feels secure about eating out with friends, going to movies, getting a massage, etc. and doesn't feel threatened about losing her motherhood if she enjoys herself. A mother who leads a fulfilling and rewarding life by taking an active interest in her field of work, relationships, society, recreation, rest, everything under the sun and pushes herself to her max potential has a good chance of being an ideal mother. Try telling any man that now he has a child, he should stop watching the IPL match, forgo that promotion at work, the badminton match in the club, not meet up with his friends and not shave and he will laugh it off. Tell him again that this has a chance of making him an ideal father and he will look the other way. Try telling a woman these things and she will buy it; we like digging our own graves. We will suppress our potential and then feel that this is it, I have a child now, I have to feel complete and not frustrated. The frustration isn't coming from the fact that looking after infants is physically demanding, it comes because we expect one act or the role of motherhood to compensate for everything we have given up on. It never can babe, it's just too unrealistic. And then because it doesn't make life "meaningful" like they say, we give up on some more and land up having a dull mind, tired body and a lingering feeling that the "real me" is lost. I mean, there is this huge sense of discontentment, like somebody cheated on us big-time, that somebody didn't give us the complete or true picture of motherhood.

'Motherhood is a huge responsibility and to successfully carry it out you need super fitness levels. You will feel fit: a) when you get good rest b) when you eat right and eat yummy food c) when you exercise d) when you get back to a healthy sex life. When a mother enjoys good fitness levels, she doesn't have to carry out a feasibility study for every small or big thing. She simply has developed the required strength in her body and flexibility in her mind to suit the new role and the responsibilities that come with it. She has the clarity in her mind that the role and responsibilities are going to change as the baby grows initially from month to month, then from year to year, and eventually the young adult may only look to her from time to time for advice or feedback and will truly appreciate being left on her/his own. The mother, however, will always remain everybody's ultimate fallback option.'

Challenging motherhood

The tea room in Windamere (a beautiful heritage hotel in Darjeeling) has vintage pictures and maps, eighteenth-century furniture, couches, a fireplace, and rays from the sunset filtering through the glass windows. Neema, the lady who serves tea, seems to have come straight out of some old

English film. The fresh 'from our private gardens' Darjeeling tea is good, but my mother apologetically asks Neema, 'Ready-made chai milega kya?' She nods yes and my mom gains the confidence to ask for more. 'Masala chai?' (not so apologetic now). 'Yes!' 'Wow!'

Meanwhile, the conversation in the room filled with goras from all over moves from trekking in Sikkim, to getting robbed in Delhi and finally settles down on a cute little one-year-old who is crawling all over (yes, there were enough women in the room). As the mother responds to all statements ranging from, 'Wow! You made it here with a one-year-old?' and 'She looks like a really manageable baby! You must be having a lot of help!' to 'Have you carried her food?' she asks her husband if he is done with his tea. He is and says he will take the baby and change her nappy and the lady can chat. A chorus 'Awwwww!' all around. The goras, the kalas, the browns and everything in between are struck with awe in the tea parlour. In a heritage room we all displayed our sadiyon ka mental conditioning. It's 'awwww' if the husband volunteers to change nappies and 'aargh' if the woman is not up to it once in a while. World over, it's the same. The colour of the skin or the fact that we come from diverse cultures doesn't seem to influence our heritage of discrimination.

Another thing, almost every woman sitting there was trying to tell this young mother that she should be grateful for the family/husband/finances that enable her to travel with her baby. How did we all overlook the fact that she must be doing more than her bit to travel with her baby, and that somebody needed to pat her back and say a word or two about her courage. How come everybody, especially us women, think and say that other women are simply luckier than us or are somehow better taken care of than us? Come on, don't we all know how much a mother has to plan just to make a trip to the garden? So the next time you find a mother braving a new country/state/district etc., tell her it's women like her who do you proud and please don't remind them that they should thank paraphernalia for support. The most supportive husband/family is helpless in the face of a woman who doesn't want to help herself or take charge of her life. As women we know that and we should never forget to acknowledge that in our words.

Post-pregnancy myths and facts

1. The maalish, the dhuan and the customary bath

If nothing else, at least these rituals give you some time off from your baby and all other responsibilities. Yes, it's important to take 'time off' from the baby. Why? To stay fresh and enthu and to keep up your motivational levels. In sports, Sachin Tendulkar, our superhero, our god, Mr Invincible, the greatest sporting legend, the best at his game, the Little Master, is also 'rested' and kept away from the game that his name has become synonymous with. Why? If he is good at it, if he is known for it, if he is the god of cricket, then why is he kept away from cricket, even for a day or a tour or a season? The answer, actually, is so that he remains the undisputed god of cricket. To get better at his game, he has to rest. Same goes for you. To remain 'good at the game of mothering' you have to be 'rested' or kept away from the baby and, so, allow yourself the indulgence of a massage and bath.

Massage also improves your circulation, helps you relax and nourishes your joints. Just ensure that you invest in a good oil and in a good maalish or massage-wali. A lot of us use massage-waalis based on recommendations and stuff, and without doubt some of them have a good knack or talent for massage. But while you are getting a massage done, if something doesn't feel right or is too hard or too painful, ask your massage-waali to stop and give your feedback right away. The same with your bath — the water should be as cold or as hot as you prefer and not what anybody else says it should be. And the dhuan and the herbs they burn actually have medicinal properties which help you relax and stimulate recovery, nourish your joints and reproductive organs, but again, buy your herbs from a trusted source. If the smoke and heat irritates you, then just STOP. Of course, before that, check that you are not standing too far away or too close to the tava; that the heat is not too strong for you; that you are burning just the right amount of herbal mixture, etc. As long as it helps you feel good, helps you relax and refreshes, don't wait for a doctor or anybody else to validate the practice. Ask your doctor for an opinion if you must — but treat it like one, and not as a fact. If you are enjoying it, don't stop just because your doctor says to!

2. The forty-day 'curfew' and staying at your mother's house
Again another misunderstood practice. This was meant to make life easy for women, not restrict them or upset family equations. Now, though, some communities impose such strict restrictions on women during this time that it does nothing but depress them. Women need to look at this forty-day period as 'me time'. This is also the time when a new mother needs maximum support and advice from a trusted elder who's 'been there, done that'. Typically, it's easier to get all this at her mother's place, but if this is not possible for some reason (say the mother is ailing), then it doesn't make sense to impose yourself on her. Stay wherever you feel you have max chance of rest and recovery, period. Don't think about it as following or defying tradition. The only tradition worth considering is the 'tradition' to maximise the new mother's chances of survival by allowing for maximum recovery, and good nourishment and love, of course.

3. The ghee, the laddoo and the works

'To eat or not to eat' — that question is bigger than 'To be or not to be'! And sorry there is no straight answer, no logic, no reason — just go by pure, simple instinct. Does it taste yummy? Does it calm your nerves? Does it energise you? Does it make you smile? Does it make you feel strong? Does it make you feel light? If you answered 'YES', eat the ghee, eat the laddoo. Use fresh produce though, make it with love, store it in secure bottles and containers (please, no plastic) and eat it responsibly. The last thing that you need right now is calorie deprivation. You need good nourishment and you need good calories (bye-bye sugar-free chocolate and fat-free cheese) because you can't afford any stupid 'dieting' right now. All that avoiding calories will do is increase fatigue levels, making you feel dull in the body, not up to changing diapers, leave alone hitting the gym. And because most diets have strict no-no foods (ghee, laddoo top the list), you will feel like a failure. Of course you will blame it on your mother or MiL, whoever forced the laddoo or ghee down your throat, but remember it's not their fault. The fault lies in the 'no-no/strictly avoid' list. Feeling like a failure and feeling dull in the body (because of low calorie intake) and having disrupted sleep at night is a ripe ground for post-partum depression, okay? So what, eat everything that they thuso in your mouth? NO! Stay sensible with everything you eat, eat often and stay light on your stomach. Only you get to decide the right quantity of food for yourself, nobody outside of you has the power to do that, not even your mother, let alone your dietician.

4. Drink milk to produce milk

As true as 'eat gulab jamuns to produce gulab jamuns'. How much milk your glands produce depends on many factors, the main one being how much your baby needs. The other main factors that influence milk production are:

a. Nutritional status: Is your body well nourished? Are you receiving adequate amounts of protein and calcium from your diet? And, as I told you earlier, you need to build your calcium banks at least a year in advance; it's not something that can be built overnight. So eat sensibly, eat fresh and eat in peace for maximum assimilation of nutrients.

b. Rest and recovery: Are you fussing and wasting energy over wasteful things (wasteful is my word: wasting time, energy and much needed nutrients) like who gave me what as a present, who said what, has the maid come, has my husband eaten, etc. Sleep well, allow yourself to be pampered, give up ideas of 'self reliance' and ask your partner, family, friends, maids for help. Be specific: Can you take a chutti and look after the baby full day and night and bring her/him to me for feeding ONLY? Please don't expect that 'At least now they should understand' and all that jazz; instead think, 'At least now I should speak my mind'.

Can you avoid milk altogether? Totally. If you don't like milk, don't force yourself. Your body is happy to assimilate nutrients and amino acids (building blocks of protein) from curd, rotis, laddoos, ghee, rice, dal, khichdi, poha, idli — everything that's taaza and made at home and made fresh (please don't eat last night's dal). So don't let yourself or others get fussy about milk. The idea is to have complete meals, those which provide wholesome nourishment, energy, vitamins, minerals and hydration.

5. Eating irresponsibly, glorifying it

Making dal rice into a paste or smashing apple for your toothless baby and then running behind her to feed her? Okay, suit yourself, if this is how you want to inculcate 'food values' in your kids. But eating what they haven't eaten? Nah, not cool. You have teeth and all other senses required to relish every flavour and aroma in food. So eat food meant for adults. The paste that you are eating gets converted to fat too, specially when your body really doesn't need it. Make food in small amounts for your baby too, and feed her only what she will happily eat. Food that you force down by fooling or distracting her won't get assimilated into her system. It won't make her stronger, taller — it will just stress her out right now and give rise to food fears later in life.

The mommy body

So it's been three-four months since you've had your baby, and you still have a little tyre around your stomach and you're heavier than normal on the scale. There are two things you should know: if you're nursing, you will land up weighing a little more because of the additional breast tissue and because of the extra fluids in your body. Also your body wants to store energy reserves because of the daily tasks of waking up early, feeding etc., so these things will tip the scales. The second thing is that there's an evolutionary reason for that little bulge around the navel — it safeguards you against all diseases and any food scarcity. It's normal, and in fact to your advantage to have this little bulge. Your body is doing its best to help you stay strong, fit, and most importantly, disease-free. So don't keep pinching your bulge saying, 'Yeh nahi gaya abhi tak.' Feel happy with your mommy body; it's your body's gift to you at this critical time of your life.

Yes, weight loss will be slower because pregnancy leads to unbelievable losses of bone density and muscle weight. You lose calcium and minerals like chromium and iron. The exercise and diet programme you adopt should help you make gains in lean body weight (which could sometimes actually mean an increase in your body weight on the scale). This is the one time when you must change your focus from total weight loss to specifically gaining lean body weight. We all want to be yummy mummies, but this can only happen if we gain all the lean body weight we've lost during pregnancy. One reason why rural women or women who get back their bodies soon after having their babies do so is because they start off with a higher lean body weight. You may not like it, but eventually you'll look slimmer than what the scales tell you.

When will you start to lose weight? When you get your first period after having a baby, it's a sign that you're biologically ready to lose weight. Also, when you stop breastfeeding, because you no longer need to store those extra fluids and your body will see no need to store that extra energy. It's a good time to remember that if you go on a crash diet you'll crash in weight, but you won't end up happy or looking yummy. So enjoy being a mommy and that mommy body for as long as it lasts.

THE FOUR STRATEGIES

Nutrition strategies	Exercise strategies	Sleep strategies	
God! Do you need more nutrition advice? Aren't you getting everything from 'eat for two'/'don't eat baingan — baby will become dark'/'don't eat this, eat that', blah blah, blah.

Let me spare you further confusion with just two important tips:

If any of the pills/ vitamins/ hormones make you feel uncomfortable, speak up and tell your doctor. There is no law that says the more painful the procedure, the more glorious the pregnancy.

Listen to yourself, more than ever. Tune into and respect your body's cues regarding food, timings, quantities — college degrees or number of pregnancies doesn't qualify anybody to tell you what to eat.

Your thyroid works overtime during pregnancy so read the chapter on the thyroid (Chapter 6) carefully. | Working out improves your and your baby's health, physically, mentally and emotionally.

If you are already pregnant, it's not a good time to try a new form of exercise. Stick to what you've been doing.

Post delivery, your body will tell you when it's ready for more action. Listen to that call and take immediate action ☺.

Seemingly easy and simple exercises can be disastrous if you don't account for the excess flexibility, loss of calcium and hormonal changes that your body goes through during and immediately after pregnancy. So seek professional help and at all times allow your body to be your teacher/trainer.

On the other hand, seemingly hardcore exercises like taekwondo, shirsasana, running etc. may be a piece of cake if you have enjoyed good fitness levels and the guidance of a competent teacher. | Sleeping is crucial for hormonal harmony, without which a healthy and safe pregnancy will remain only a dream.

During pregnancy the last thing you should do is eat a dessert before bedtime — all it does is it piles inches around the waist and upsets nutrient delivery to the foetus.

Post pregnancy, how much you enjoy your motherhood and your baby depends on how well you sleep in the nights.

Recovering from the delivery, production of milk and beating post-partum blues is all delicately balanced on the quality of your sleep. So give yourself at least two nights a week when you can sleep uninterrupted during the night. Either express your milk or have husband/ family bring the baby to you only for feeding — not for nappy change and other stuff. | If marriage makes you secondary to the husband, then motherhood puts you in third place (if not lower) in your order of priorities.

Kids whose mothers are strong, happy and calm make the most of their childhood and life. For this to happen, mommy's got to be No. 1 on her own priority list.

Unconditional love, the ability to endlessly give comes easy to a mother — biological or adopted is irrelevant.

Give yourself and your baby time to bloom as individuals so that you make a rocking team. Even when she is forty and you are touching seventy.

If in your enthu of being an 'ideal' mother you forget that you exist, then you are in for a 'real' rude shock.

Accept and make time to nurture your body who gave you this beautiful baby. Don't insult her by pinching at various places or by calling her fat. |

Real life diet analysis

*Vaishali Sawant is a thirty-four-year-old working mother of two
(in fact, she is a nursing mother), juggling between her household
responsibilities and work (quite clichéd, isn't it?).*

She lives in Dubai, and is a Marathi mulgi married to a south Indian.
She feels her pregnancies (both delivered through C-section) have
majorly contributed to her flabby body.

This is how she got in touch with me:

Dear Rujuta Ma'am,

*Been curious about your 'technique' ever since Kareena Kapoor's
fantastic physique became a matter of national interest. Then my
brother (who has an IISA certificate and is a complete fitness freak)
sent me your book 'Don't Lose Your ...'. Needless to say, the book
hooked me completely. No diet or health book has made so much sense
to me.*

*I am thirty-four years old and have so far never done anything on
a committed basis to take care of my body. While I have overall good
habits (lots of water, regular meals, no soft or fizzy drinks, no alcohol,
no smoking or late-night partying), two pregnancies have made me
quite tired and flabby.*

*Throughout my life I have never been a sporty person and the only
exercise I truly enjoy is walking. After my first son was almost one
year old, I replaced my office lunch with two salads (1 sprouts bhel
and 1 soya beans misal) and quickly lost weight. Everyone said how
good I looked — but my stomach and arms remained soft and untoned
(also because I did no exercise).*

*By the time I conceived my second baby, I had gone from 55 kgs to
58 kgs and then through my pregnancy put on about 20 kgs more. I
am about 66 kgs now. I have already started putting your principles
in practice, but need your specific inputs as now and for the rest of
my life, I don't want to be just thin and look good — I want to be
strong, lean and toned. I have dreams of trekking to Manasarovar,
white water rafting (am taking swimming lessons) and running at least
1 marathon.*

Look forward to starting this journey with you.

Three-day diet recall

Time	Food/Drink	Activity Recall	Workout
Day 1			
6.40 a.m.		Got up just in time to say bye to son as he left for school. Usually husband gets him ready in the morning. If he is travelling, I wake up at 6 a.m. and get him ready	
6.45 – 7.00 a.m.		Changed baby's nappy, made 1 feed for her and took her to the garden for a brief stroll	
7.00 – 9.00 a.m.	1 cup tea (Red Label Nature Cure + milk + sugar) and 1 chapatti	Made breakfast for husband, packed dabba and snacks for him, told the maid what veggies to cut for lunch. Sat with husband as he had his breakfast. Sterilised equipment for pumping breast milk	
8.30 a.m.	2 idlis and some coconut chutney, after some time 1 rawa laddoo, also 1 small glass of leftover protein shake (made for husband with orange juice and 1 scoop of whey protein)		
9.00 to 9.30 a.m.		Read newspaper, checked mail (while waiting for baby to wake up from her nap)	
9.30 – 10.15 a.m.		Gave baby a bath, took a bath and did puja	

Time	Food	Activity	
10.15 – 10.30 a.m.		Called boss and discussed work-related issues	
10.30 a.m.	1 bowl of channa and roasted peanuts		
10.30 a.m. – 12 p.m.		Worked on laptop	
12.15 p.m.	1 bowl of rice, prawn curry and some soya bean granules sabzi, 1 bowl of curd with a bit of sugar	Pumped breast milk, waited for son to come home from school while watching TV	
1.05 to 1.40 p.m.	I make it a point to drink at least 3 litres of water every day. So I fill up a 1.5 litre bottle (refill it by mid-day) and keep it with me, wherever I go, whatever I do — I keep sipping	Went out to pick son up as bus dropped him off, washed him and changed his clothes, checked his dabba and school bag and gave him lunch	
1.40 – 2.50 p.m.		Read a magazine in bed and took a nap	
3.00 p.m.		Started working again. While working, also supervised son's homework	
3.30 – 5.30 p.m.	1 cup tea (Red Label Nature Cure + milk + sugar) and 1 chapatti	Multitasked between working, feeding baby, playing with son and baby, sending son to swimming class	
5.30 – 6.15 p.m.		Gave baby a bath and then son a bath. Sat with son while he had his dinner	
7.00 p.m.	1 chapatti, 1 bowl of dal and some beans sabzi and 1 rawa laddoo		

7.30 – 8.00 p.m.		Brushed son's teeth, got him ready for bed, read him a story and put him to sleep	
8.10 – 9.15 p.m.			Went for a 3.5 km walk. Normally I walk about 7 kms in 1 hour. But today met a friend and walked very slowly with her
9.15 – 10.15 p.m.		Took a shower, watched TV with hubby while pumping breast milk	
9.30 p.m.	1 bowl of dal and a little bit of prawn curry, then 1 small piece of chocolate cake		
10.15 – 11.00 p.m.		Woke up baby, changed her nappy, fed her and put her to sleep	
11.00 – 11.30 p.m.		Read a bit and went to sleep	
12 a.m.		Woke up as son was crying in his room, put him to sleep in his dad's room	
3 a.m.		Woke up with a bad sinus cold. Took 1 Allegra	
3.00 to 3.45 a.m.		Nursed baby and put her to sleep	
Day 2			
7.25 a.m.		Woke up and went down to kitchen	
7.30 a.m.	1 cup tea (Red Label Nature Cure + milk + sugar) and 1 chapatti		

7.35 – 8.30 a.m.		Made dabba for hubby, told maid what to make for lunch, sterilised breast pump equipment, made feed for baby	
8.30 a.m.	2 peserattus (green moong dosa) and a little bit of coconut chutney		
8.45 a.m.		Fed baby	
9.00 – 10.00 a.m.		Bathed baby, took a bath, did puja and pumped milk. Started work on laptop	
11.30 a.m.	1 bowl of channa and roasted peanuts		
12.15 p.m.	1 bowl of rice, chicken dhania curry and 1 rawa laddoo		
12.30 – 2.00 p.m.		Multi-tasked between working, receiving son from school and serving him lunch and then back to my laptop	
2.15 p.m.	1 slice of chocolate cake	Had a friend over, who came to visit my baby	
3.00 – 4.15 p.m.		Took a nap	
4.20 p.m.	1 cup of tea		
4.30 p.m.		Dropped son to art class and then dropped in for a friend's tea party	
5.00 p.m.	(At tea party) 1 bowl of dahi vada, fruit salad and 2 shammi kababs		

5.30 – 6.30 p.m.		Went and picked up son from class and brought him home. Gave him and baby a bath, made feed for baby	
6.30 – 7.30 p.m.		Alternated between sitting with son for dinner and putting baby to sleep	
7.15 p.m.	Half a cup of milk with a little sugar and Horlicks (leftover by son)		
7.30 – 8.45 p.m.		Went to supermarket to get groceries	
8.45 – 9.00 p.m.		Took a bath and changed into nightclothes	
9.10 p.m.	2 slices of bread, chicken curry, curds with sugar and 2 slices of mango		
9.30 – 10.45 p.m.		Worked on laptop	
11.00 p.m.		Woke up baby, changed her nappy and fed her	
11.30 p.m.		Went to sleep	
Day 3 (Holiday)			
6.10 – 7.00 a.m.		Woke up, changed baby's nappy, fed her and took her down to play with her brother	
7.00 a.m.	1 cup tea (Red Label Nature Cure + milk + sugar) and 1 chapatti		
7.00 – 7.30 a.m.		Chatted with family, gave son breakfast, got ready for swimming class	

7.20 a.m.	1 banana		
7.45 a.m.		Went to swimming class	
8.00 – 9.00 a.m.			Went swimming
9.00 – 9.15 a.m.		Showered, changed and took son for his swimming class	
9.35 a.m.	1 granola bar		
10.00 a.m.		Brought son back home	
10.30 a.m.	1 banana and then some peanuts	Made a snack for son, cooked lunch	
11.00 a.m. – 12 p.m.		Gave bath to baby, took bath and did puja. Expressed milk	
12.00 p.m.	2 chapattis, methi and matar sabzi and dal		
12.30 – 2.00 p.m.		Played with son and baby and chatted with hubby	
2.00 – 3.30 p.m.		Took a nap	
3.45 p.m.	1 cup tea (Red Label Nature Cure + milk + sugar) and 1 chapatti	Worked on laptop	
4.30 p.m.	1 cup tea and some peanut butter		
5.30 – 6.10 p.m.			Went for a brisk walk. Did 3.5 kms in 30 minutes!
6.10 – 7.30 p.m.		Gave baby a bath, took a bath, fed baby and put her to sleep	
7.30 – 8.00 p.m.		Made a salad for husband and made arrangements for next day's cooking	

8.00 p.m.	1 chapatti, egg curry (1 egg), dal and salad		
8.30 – 10.00 p.m.		Worked on laptop	
10.00 p.m.		Expressed milk	
10.30 p.m.		Changed baby's nappy, fed her and put her to sleep	
11.00 p.m.		Went to sleep	

Evaluation of the recall

Vaishali's recall actually reasserted my belief that women have an inborn talent to multitask! Phew!! How did she manage to do so many things in the day, with not even a minute to breathe!

From her recall it's easy to see that most of Vaishali's activities revolve around her three-month-old baby, son and husband (in this order of priority at the moment). Except for an hour's walk/swim and half an hour reading in the day, she didn't have any time for herself!

She believes her weight gain is caused just by 'post pregnancy, C-section'. In fact, she had put on close to twenty-four kilos during her second pregnancy (as compared to the 'normal' ten–fifteen kilos) — all due to 'pregnancy-induced bingeing', soaring sweet cravings and lack of exercise.

Vaishali was following the four principles mentioned in *Don't Lose Your Mind, Lose Your Weight* and was trying to eat every two hours. But what she didn't realise was that her requirements were much more (almost double) than what she was providing her body.

Pregnancy is a stage in a woman's life when she needs to nourish herself as well as her foetus (but this is what happens — a state of malnourishment for the mother and complete nourishment of the foetus). Whatever is your food/nutrient intake during this period, most of it gets used up for the nourishment of your foetus. It is necessary to meet your body's increased requirements so that there is equal distribution of nutrients to the mother as well as the foetus. If the mother is deprived of the necessary nutrients (which happens in most cases), it leads to faster ageing (the body ages by four years with a loss in the lean body mass) and creates a stressful environment in the body. All this eventually leads to the deposition of fat stores (nutrient deprivation — putting the body in starvation/stressful mode) and a lowering of your lean body stores (muscle mass + bone mineral stores).

So post pregnancy is the time when your body is actually working on rebuilding all your nutrient and lean body stores (so your body is in a high metabolic state). Your body is overworking because it doesn't just have to improve your nutrient stores, but also the nutrient quality and quantity of breast milk (poor nutritional status of the mother = poor breast milk secretion = poor nutritional status of the baby).

What was happening in Vaishali's case is that, even though she was trying to eat every two hours and had taken up an activity in the day (swimming/brisk walking), her mind was not in sync with her body. The food that she was eating was not nourishing her as she was continuously worried about her baby, expressing breast milk, feeding her older son, sitting with him for his homework, packing dabbas for husband and son, changing nappies, dropping her son for classes, fetching him, grocery shopping … the list was endless.

She just needed to calm down, tone down all her energies and responsibilities at home and work, and distribute her household work with her husband — especially looking after her little baby and changing her nappies in the middle of the night. Vaishali just needed to sleep, rest and recover!

Modifications

Vaishali's plan of action was to eat right, nourish and pamper her body, pay her body enough attention to understand its requirements, exercise regularly and sleep on time (let her body recover).

Post pregnancy, if the body receives the right nutrients and is well nourished, it becomes very easy for it to get rid of the fat stores which develop during pregnancy (on account of poor nutrient supply during pregnancy). The body needs a lot more recovery to cope with internal organ functions (digestion, respiration) as well as external day-to-day activities and exercise (Vaishali's endless list of activities through the day).

Vaishali just needed to let her body feel loved, cared for, well-fed and well-nourished (just like she wanted it for her baby ☺).

Although she was managing her daily chores, it was leaving her tired and completely exhausted by the end of the day. She needed to improve on her energy levels to keep her going through the day with ease. She needed to start with regular workouts as well, especially weight-training, to improve on her lean body stores (which would improve her body composition and further lower her fat stores).

She can modify her diet as follows:

Meal 1 (7.00 a.m.): Protein shake (needed it to start off her day and let her body recover from the overnight fast)

Meal 2 (8.00 a.m.): 2 egg whites + whole wheat toast (easy to prepare in the mornings, while she is struggling with packing dabbas, feeding her baby, all other early-morning household chores)

Meal 3 (10.00 a.m.): Fruit yogurt (for her sweet tooth ☺)

Meal 4 (12.00 p.m.): Rice + fish curry + veggies (as she loved fish and this was a good time for her to eat her meal in peace)

Meal 5 (2.00 p.m.): Peanuts (another of her favourites)

Meal 6 (4.00 p.m.): Veg sandwich with cheese or homemade nashta

Meal 7 (6.00 p.m.): Chapatti + dal + sabzi

Meal 8 (8.00 p.m.): Stir-fry veggies with olives (7-8) or dal + sabzi

Meal 9 (10.00 p.m.): ½ scoop protein shake in milk (needed it again for an overnight recovery)

Vaishali needed to improve her carb, protein and essential fat stores, as well as vitamin B stores (particularly B6 and B12), Omega-3 fatty acids, vitamins A, C and E and antioxidants (with selenium, zinc, chromium) — all of which would improve her body's recovery and also improve the nutrient density/quality of her breast milk. She also needed calcium to replenish the body's bone mineral stores.

Vaishali modified her eating pattern as given and also started weight-training regularly. She saw that her relationship with her baby and son improved as well (they were loving their new energetic, chirpy mom ☺).

Her husband too stepped up and took on the responsibility of looking after their baby in the night (they mutually decided on equally splitting nights). This helped Vaishali catch up with her long-lost sleep as well ☺.

5

Menopause — Coming Of Age

Menopause — finally, the coming of age for women. We spend our lives as if our biology has cursed our fate or written our destiny, leading lives that have been limited, or at least influenced, by our roles of wife and mother. Now that we won't get our periods, will we ever be able to bear a child? Wait! Would anybody even have married us if we weren't chumming? I mean, without our monthly cycle, aren't we exactly like men? Is it our journey towards becoming a man, or is it a journey where we can explore womanhood beyond our biology and hormones?

Real life example
'All my life, all I wanted and wished for was my periods to end. I got mine when I was in ninth standard, very late by today's standards, but I was glad to have them as late as possible, and not have them at all, if that was possible. And then all through my teens and early twenties, I wanted them to disappear and hoped that I could get menopause right now! When my mother heard me say that once, she slapped me and said nobody would marry me even if my periods were irregular so forget about not having them. Having an unmarried daughter at home was the biggest curse, was her funda. Then I got married and we "planned" (used contraceptives)

for two years. Then do saal ke baad, I stopped using the pill, and for two years struggled to get pregnant. My mom-in-law would cry every month that I got my periods after the third year of my shaadi. Not being able to bear a child was the biggest curse for a woman, was *her* funda. Between these two fundas, my life just went on and today, with my kids grown up, my mom gone and mom-in-law sick, I am super lost. I hated the pain and pads every month, but now that I am close to, in fact, almost post-menopause, I've not had my periods for four months, I am lost. I don't know what to do. I feel ... I don't know. I can't tell you. I am like one pendulum oscillating between "I have found myself" — no responsibilities, no periods — to "I am lost", I am no longer a woman. I must be a special case na? Have any of your clients ever said this to you before?'

Yes, they've said all this, and felt worse. But the thing is that only my clients who are younger and expecting menopause have said and felt worse. The ones who have reached and left menopause behind them are at total peace with the process. Speculation about what is coming next never ends in a woman's life. **Our body is like a blind curve on the high Himalayan roads.** What will the next turn bring? A beautiful meadow, with bright yellow flowers? Huge snow-clad mountains, with their peaks hidden under the clouds? You just never know what's coming next, or how to cope with it. One moment you are in school hearing stories about what happens in your first period and having nightmares over it — will I bleed to death? Next moment you are having nightmares about what will happen the first time you have sex —

will it hurt horribly? Next moment you are pregnant and every month your stomach is changing and the baby is kicking, you are dying to deliver, but you are thinking — are they going to shave my hair off and cut my vagina to allow the baby's head to pass? Will they stitch me up after that and how much will it hurt? Then post-forty, every minor change in your monthly period, you speculate. Is this it? Is it finally over? Will my uterus collapse? Will I grow a moustache? Will I develop osteoporosis? And how will I cope with hot flushes?

And what is valid and true of every phase of a woman's life, through her constantly changing hormonal environment, is valid and true for menopause too: 'It's not all that bad; in fact, it's really okay.' But just like our first period, we are scared and speculative before we reach menopause. And just like menarche (the date on which you get your first period or onset of menstruation — so it's the exact opposite of menopause), we have little or no information or education on how to deal with this phase. It's not discussed openly, remains a taboo subject, and at best we have access to other people's speculation or hear tales of what happened to somebody's mother/ aunt/friend. Now if we start anticipating that our menopause will be like somebody else's or like one of the many stories (nightmares) we have heard, we could be *so* wrong. Menopause, in many ways, is like marriage: every woman has a unique one. **How difficult or smooth your menopause will be depends on a variety of factors, not the least of which is your nutritional status.** If you have been working out for the last ten years or more, eating right, sleeping on time and enjoy good fitness levels, you will be able to celebrate menopause as a natural progression of the journey called life.

A woman who enjoys or feels in control of her body is typically the type who has learnt to take responsibility of her well-being, both physically and mentally. She is so in tune with her body, mind and senses, that she has both the intelligence and sensibility to understand that menopause is not a disease or a condition, it is a natural phenomenon. What comes naturally to the body shouldn't be feared or made a big deal out of, it should only be understood and accepted (celebrated).

Why me?

This is a question that plagues many a woman's life: why me? Why should I be the only one adjusting every time? Why should I compromise on this, *again*? Why must I get my periods every month? Why can I not eat with others while menstruating? Why should I leave my mom's house and move to my husband's parents' place, and not the other way round? Why should I be the one to make the chai, even if I'm tired after returning from work? Why should I be the one who gets pregnant? Why should I change my name/surname after marriage? Why should I wake up and feed the baby while my husband snores? Why should I be blamed if my son loses weight during his vacation? Why can I not live with the man I love? Why is it my responsibility to keep the kitchen clean? Why must I not ask 'all these' questions? Why must I menopause? … Feel free to add to my list.

Most questions go unasked, as we fear asking them even to ourselves. The ones that get asked go unanswered or get the age-old answer — aisa hi hote aa raha hai or yehi hamara riwaaaz hai, or worse, women have to adjust if they want peace at home. Pure, unadulterated nonsense. Is it really our tradition, custom, culture to impose restrictions, limitations, boundaries for women? Can a peaceful home environment truly be achieved only after ensuring that

---

women's lives are compromised on? Are we really such a regressive and unequal society, or is it plain misunderstood and misinterpreted customs, traditions and rituals? Shouldn't we have the good sense and courage to re-evaluate and review our belief system? By not asking questions, especially those related to biases (beliefs) against our hormones, biology and gender, we show complete disrespect towards our body, our intelligence, nature, tradition, religion, culture and divinity itself.

Nature to the rescue

Nature has taken special care of its female species, especially those of the human form because nature perceives us as special, intelligent and important enough to be protected and nurtured, and wants to go out of its way to allow us to thrive and lead fulfilling, meaningful lives. That's exactly why it created or 'selected' menopause. Could nature be wrong? (No, but are we hell-bent on proving otherwise, yeah, in all probability.) Here's what nature had in mind: the human female species has a large cost (nutritionally, physically, emotionally) associated with fertility, reproduction and ensuring survival of the offspring or newborn. There has to be some physiological and biological mechanism to curtail fertility and reproduction (to ensure good health and survival of the mother and the existing offspring) — hmm how about introducing menopause, cessation of the menstrual cycle?

Maybe Mother Nature also had the insight (she is not called a mother for nothing) that eventually we would lose our ability to be assertive about our rights and responsibilities towards our vagina and womb. She probably knew that it was easy for the human female species to be clouded, emotional, brainwashed about her reproductive rights through religion, tradition, custom or some equally flimsy grounds. That the highly sensitive, emotional, intuitive nature of a woman (due to the hormonal environment) was like a double-edged sword and there was a huge possibility that the sword would hurt/claim the woman as the first victim if not used well. With proper training and nurturing though, a woman would feel empowered to use her emotional, sensitive and intuitive nature to take intelligent, reasonable and smart decisions for herself, her offspring and her environment. But it was too risky to assume that every woman would learn to use the sword or her nature (now popularly described as complex and complicated) to her advantage/ for the greater good. So menopause is nature's brilliant back-up option — you get to enjoy sex (hopefully you have learnt to) and you stay protected from pregnancies and nursing and everything else that comes with it.

My great grandmother (Appa's mother) gave birth to not one, five or ten but seventeen children. Appa was her third child and she still had enough nutrients left in her to pass on to her foetus and offspring. She also still had interest in children. Married off at the age of eight or nine years with little or no education, she was not really in a position to understand what 'reproductive rights' meant. However, she suffered from everything that one can suffer from when one is not aware of one's rights. It's not that my great grandfather had some agenda against her or that he was a terrible man; he was as much a victim of her not asserting her right to say no. My great grandmother had been trained to think that she shouldn't deny her husband anything at all, including sex of course. And so one after another they had seventeen children. She paid a much bigger price because it took a toll on her physically. It drained my beautiful, bright, chirpy great grandmother. Her first eleven children survived into adulthood; amongst them, the first four siblings enjoyed better protection from diseases and other infections rampant during their childhood. The other children remained vulnerable to frequent infections and even today, in their late fifties and sixties, are not as energetic or fit as the older siblings. Children twelve to seventeen were the really tough part, specially for the siblings, as they witnessed their younger brothers and sisters dying either within a few hours of their birth or succumbing to various diseases like plague even before they turned two. How did your mother take all this? I asked Appa. She was too busy filling water, cooking and feeding her dozen children, so tired that she didn't have the privilege to mourn or get depressed about the illnesses and deaths of her own children, he replied. One of her children was born after my mother was born, something that she was really embarrassed about: that her daughter-in-law and she were pregnant at the same time. Luckily menopause came to her rescue and prevented further pregnancies and embarrassment for her. It's also for women in situations like my great grandmother that menopause exists.

Nature has the wisdom to understand that a woman's energies are better directed towards caring and nurturing her existing offspring so that it improves their fitness and survival (also hers) instead of directing them to producing more offspring that takes a toll on her health and reduces the chances of survival and the good health of the younger ones.

There is a hypothesis that a grandmother is crucial to ensure the good health and survival of her grandchildren. This is especially true in 'bad times', whether during natural disasters like floods, famines and earthquakes, or emotionally-charged situations like bad marriages, separation, divorces, violent marriages, etc. With menopause, a grandmother can direct her energies to meaningful pursuits of life including looking after her grandchildren. Without menopause, our grandmothers would still be busy carrying out the responsibilities of being a wife and mother and therefore be too exhausted for her grandchildren. My great grandmother was too exhausted for her grandchildren and understandably so. Here's another interesting titbit — maternal grandmothers improve the survival chances of existing offspring, while paternal grandmothers improve the birth rate of offspring. Ah! Complicated.

Healthy ovaries — healthy menopause

Enough masala. Now what's important to understand is that our ovaries go through a change and therefore the hormones change too. An ovum is the largest cell in the human body; the sperm is the smallest (surprising, considering who does the most dadagiri!). To fertilise just one egg, the male has to send millions of sperms. It's almost like women were the smarter lot, choosing Sri Krishna and allowing the men to think that they got a better deal by getting Krishna's entire army. An unarmed Krishna refusing to do anything other than guiding Arjun's chariot is a thousand times more valuable than a fully-equipped army of millions, right?

With time, the size of the ovaries starts decreasing and so does the production of hormones. As long as you have your ovaries (they can be removed surgically), your menopause can be a smooth transition. The key really is to keep the ovaries healthy (receiving good blood circulation). For this you will need to ensure that your diet remains nutritionally rich and make exercise an important part of your life. Regular exercise keeps the waist slim and prevents it from thickening. A thicker waist makes you prone to a host of lifestyle diseases like high blood pressure, diabetes, heart disease, weaker bones, joints, etc. Remember the thing we learnt about waist-to-hip ratio (Chapter 3)? The bigger danger than gaining weight around menopause is the change in the fat distribution. The only sensible thing to do then is to keep your lifestyle in check and allow the hormones to go through their natural transition and the balance they are trying to achieve. Your ovaries work hard for you all their life; at this crucial juncture, all that they expect is that you provide them with a stable environment to carry out a smooth transition to menopause.

One of the reasons that fertility drops just before you reach menopause is to allow you to lead a more stable and healthy lifestyle. Think about it, if you were to have a child just before menopause, then you would be staying up nights and feeding. Late nights, whether it's for nursing or partying, reduce your body's ability to recover and change your hormonal balance, specifically that of your insulin. With small children or babies around, women typically become indifferent to their own nutritional needs. And a poor nutritional status makes a smooth menopause impossible. At a time when the body is allowing you a chance to restore your calcium levels and bone density before hitting menopause, you will instead be focusing on feeding your babies, even if you are starving yourself.

Having children around also makes it difficult for women to spare the time for exercise: just the 'normal' job of bringing them up, answering their questions and keeping up with their energy levels leaves women too drained out to exercise. Lack of exercise results in lack of circulation and oxygenation to the ovaries (blood supply and oxygen), again making it difficult for them to go through their natural process of menopause.

Nature works with us and creates conditions for us to have a perfectly smooth menopause. The problem here is, we don't quite support nature's work. Most women gain weight post thirty either because they've just had a baby, or because of a basic indifference towards getting fitter and stronger, making it difficult for their hormones to find a natural balance. Also, many women put themselves through hajjar diet and weight-loss plans, farms and fads before hitting menopause (ironically, sometimes in the hope of an easier menopause), which destroys their nutritional balance, especially that of the all-important calcium, vitamins D and B12. Most women have still to learn the benefits of sleeping on time, so they are still adjusting to the noise and sound of the TV in the bedroom, or allowing themselves to go through the emotional atyachar of our (mostly) regressive serials on TV. If women work towards their menopause like nature does, it will not become a phase where you gain weight, are prone to high blood pressure, heart disease, vaginal dryness, osteoporosis, hot flushes, sleepless nights, etc., but a natural, smooth and much-needed progression towards a healthier, meaningful and insightful existence, a brilliant chance to go beyond roles typified by biology and hormones.

Strong aur sundar

My window at Windamere overlooked the Chowrasta, the most happening place in all of Darjeeling. The Chowrasta has it all — bookshops, ice cream stalls, outdoor cafés, stores selling Darjeeling tea in all varieties (first flush, second flush), internet cafés, Tibetan artecraft shops, photographers who will click your picture and prod shy honeymooners to look, or worse, touch each other. My mom and I stared at the Chowrasta (I, between writing, and mom continuously) throughout the day, till we fell off to sleep. But what really made the Chowrasta so spectacular and addictive and central to our stay in Darjeeling was the people.

The Chowrasta is lined with benches all through and the most interesting part is that they are always occupied, *always*. From 5 a.m. till dark. Students, senior citizens, young boys and girls, not so young men and women, really old men and women, but always more women than men. In other cities, every naka/chowk/mohalla/village square/tea shop/ nukkad or any hanging out/chilling place is always dominated exclusively by men. Not in Darjeeling. It's just so therapeutic to actually watch women of all age groups sitting with other women and some men on those benches for hours together, talking, laughing, chatting or just simply doing nothing. 'Chilling or doing nothing' is almost an exclusive privilege of the 'fair and handsome' class.

But the most interesting women in the Chowrasta are the ones who work as chaiwalas and ghodawalas. And every chaiwali, no jokes, is super well-dressed. Some in jeans and shiny tops, some in traditional Tibetan wear, some in sarees, all of them without exception with rosy cheeks, pouty lips, flowers in the hair and completely celebrating womanhood. They make chai behind the railings and then jump over the railings to serve chai, bend down to pick up their glasses, chat, flirt and guide their regular and irregular tourist customers and generally have a gala time while they make their money, and of course work hard. Sandhya, the girl we drank our chai from, would trek an hour to and from her house to Chowrasta, carrying about two tiffins with her. The rest of her meals she bought from friends in Chowrasta, and worked daily from 5 a.m. to 8 p.m. nonstop.

The ghodawalis, again with all the solah shringar, kajal in their eyes, beautiful dresses depending on which tribe/community they belonged to, rode and reined in their horses with the vigour of Salman Khan in a Hindi movie. They would pick up little kids, raising them above their heads and plonking them on the horse, and then run the 1.5 kilometre 'round' around the Chowrasta. Hmm, yes, they helped the soft podgy honeymooning husbands with equal ease, lifting them, helping them on and off the horse. So much for strong and sundar, like an irritating plywood ad I saw pasted over every bus stop and hoarding in Mumbai. The 'sundar' was a girl in a figure-skating dress, petite and pretty; behind her stood a guy flexing his biceps depicting 'strong'. Come to Darjeeling, strong and sundar coexist, beautifully. Ah, one more thing, all these women look super fit and super petite. Strength doesn't mean a bulky or manly body.

Life after menopause

Most of us lead lives limited by our hormones, and menopause forces us to think beyond these limitations. Our periods have ceased but we still exist. It is nature holding up a mirror to you: look, your life is beyond a role limited to being a wife, mother or a particular gender. Overcome your limitations and soar above all the horizons you set for yourself. To help you go beyond biology, it changes your hormonal environment. **A lot of women feel angry and irritable around menopause, even the most gentle, caring and loving women**. What's the reason? Blame it on hormones? No, *thank* your hormones. The body creates a hormonal situation by weaning off progesterone and estrogen, which makes it difficult for women to succumb to the conditioning that beliefs should not be questioned. Most women will start questioning their existence, their contribution, their marriage, their motherhood, their work, careers, the meaning of life itself. The shift in hormones makes us insightful and empowers us to question everything we have lived by. If we have led limited lives because of our periods (if you remember from Chapter 2, the time when you start thinking of yourself as a girl versus a child; when you learn to laugh softly not loudly, to not jump from walls, when you learn to be less confident or assertive and slowly accept that you will always have self-doubt and start living by biases and beliefs about what you should do to become a 'good, cultured girl'), then menopause looks you in the face and says — Hey! There is life beyond this!! Grow up now!!!

Women tend to feel irritable that they may have made mindless adjustments and compromises, may feel angry that they have not done justice to their potential, that they have hardly lived for themselves, and depressed about not having lived life to its fullest. There is nothing wrong in feeling irritable, angry, depressed, really. Life is meant to be fulfilling in every role we take on, including that of wife and mother, and it's never too late (or early) to start living your life on your terms or to start doing things that will make life more meaningful, enjoyable and interesting. The insight that one gains during menopause finally allows a woman to understand that living life on her terms doesn't mean she will create havoc in anybody else's life. Living life on one's own terms is about making choices with a full understanding of consequences and having the strength to live with those choices. A new experience for many women because they mostly have their parents, in-laws, husbands, children making choices for them.

It's important for women to learn to sort out their emotions before hitting menopause. We need to have some kind of training which allows us to direct our anger, frustration, guilt, depression, irritability in a constructive manner so that it allows our personality to bloom as a wholesome individual. We are not meant to stand in the kitchen and cry; standing in the living room and shouting is just as good, as long as we start doing something about it. It's like this: complain or do something about it. Menopause and all the emotions and questions that it comes with create an environment conducive to spiritual progress in women. More and more women feel empowered to leave behind the comforts and limitations of the four walls of their home and explore the world beyond. It's not unusual for women who have always travelled with their husband and children to go on a holiday alone for the first time in their life around menopause. Or for women who have never thought beyond their own children to all of a sudden want to adopt a school and contribute in some way, or even to start their own ventures, spend money on something they always wanted or even wanting to divorce and move out of the house.

The Pushpa aunty group

GP invariably has more women than men travelling with him on his 'Connect with Himalaya' trips (enviable, na?). He is discovering that more and more women love travelling on their own whether they are single, married or mothers. His favourite, however, is what he calls the 'Pushpa aunty group'. Pushpa aunty is a wonderful woman with a grandson who is twenty years old. Two years ago, she and her gang of girls (ages ranging from fifty to seventy) discovered the joys of connecting with themselves and the Himalaya without husband, children and grandchildren in tow. Travelling with family still means carrying the baggage of your role as wife — kya khaenge dinner mein and all that. These women travel to completely off-beat places with GP and turn into giggly, chirpy, naughty little girls while on trips. On a recent trip to Chitkul, the last Indian village before the Tibet border in Kinnaur, they were at their adventurous best. They trekked from Chitkul to the last ITBP post before the border (no mean feat because Chitkul is at 3400m, high enough for altitude sickness to set in) along the Sangla river. While trekking, they met a jawan who was on his way to the post too. 'Mataji abhi bahut dur hai, aap nahi chal payegi,' he said to the group of aunties. 'Hum aa rahe hai, aap sab ko bol ke rakho and we are carrying a gift for you guys.' We are not allowed to accept gifts, said the jawan. It's something you won't be able to refuse, said the women. So some two hours of challenging walking later, they reached the post and were greeted with a standing ovation, coffee and bhajjiya by the officers. The officers couldn't refuse their gift too: they had carried a CD of Rehman's *Ma tujhe salaam,* and said this is our 'salaam' to you for guarding our borders. The officers and aunties then sang *Vande mataram* together, each one of them overwhelmed by love and emotion.

Pushpa aunty made her first trip alone at sixty, and that was to the Himalaya. So can you. The question is, are you ready to embark on the journey to explore the realms of your inner world? Are you ready to get connected with the real you?

Menopause makes it impossible for us to not see the impermanence of body, relationships and of all things around us. It is this impermanence that drives women in the quest for something more permanent, for solid truths to live by. It's for this very reason that vanaprasthashram, a phase according to the Vedantic way of life, forced women out of grihasthashram and finally into sanyashram around the time of menopause. Menopause, or rather perimenopause (around the time of menopause), is the best time for women to explore both the outside and inside worlds.

So the next time you feel angry or irritable, don't let anybody or yourself brush it aside as 'just menopause'. Know that it could be a part of exploring your inside world, it could be a clue to your suppressed emotions, suppressed anger. You could have gotten angry or upset at a seemingly small thing, but the root cause will be something bigger. Allow yourself to explore it. Writing down your niggling thoughts (no matter how seemingly irrelevant — haven't learnt sitar, etc.) gives you a chance to understand yourself and fulfil your wishes. For us to fear knowing who we are or what we would like to be or how we would like to live our life, is a complete waste of this brilliant chance that nature bestows. Btw, this is true of PMS 'irritability' too. If you pay close attention, you probably always get angry about the same thing. Instead of brushing it off as 'PMS', write it down and sort it out. We are all powerful enough to change our life and to become the person we really want to be. And you know what, channelising our efforts to be the person we want to be actually allows us to sleep well at night. So now you know all the stories of mood swings, irritability and sleepless nights are just misinterpretations of nature's blessings.

Strength and flexibility ratio

Biomechanically, our lumbar spine, i.e. what is commonly called the lower back, is vulnerable and always at the risk of injury if we have an imbalance in the strength and flexibility in the muscles around the lower back area. To maintain the good health of the spine, you need to have flexibility and the strength to bear that flexibility. For example, you may be flexible enough to reach out for something, but your muscles don't have the corresponding strength to bear that extension. Most lower-back injuries are because of a lack of strength in the area. It's that ache that comes from standing on heels, or in the kitchen, or at the end of a tiring day. It's not a slip disc, or a disc prolapse, it's a weak lower back. Women who complain about a lower back pain are typically put through an X-ray, and then an MRI and the results only state 'age-related degenerative issues'. It's basically just not enough strength as compared to flexibility and women with this pain are put on strengthening programmes. The long-term plan should be to lose weight and to strengthen the abdomen and the hip muscles — essentially build strength around the area of the spine.

The spine starts from the base of the brain, and is really considered to be like an extension of the brain, a smaller brain. So like we need both strength and flexibility in our spine, if we don't have a mind that is as strong as it is flexible, we have imbalances. It's not uncommon for women above forty to experience depression or sleeplessness or periods of big lows, and for younger women to have rash mood swings or tantrums. Women are brought up to be flexible and adaptable, not to be strong in their mind. But our mind won't be healthy if we don't have the strength corresponding to the flexibility.

You'll reach a point where the big decisions you made, where there was more flexibility than strength or the other way round, will cause you trouble. When a woman realises at forty that she didn't want to move house, that she didn't want to adjust to a particular situation, or be flexible for the entire family, she'll snap one day. She doesn't have the strength to keep up with the flexibility. So, be as strong as you are flexible. One without the other is not so much wrong as it is incomplete. There can be real flexibility only with a strong mind or a strong body.

THE FOUR STRATEGIES

Nutrition strategies	Exercise strategies	Sleep strategies	Relationship strategies
Appetite, food likes and dislikes may change as a response to the changing hormonal environment. Make peace with it, don't fuss.	If you have spent time playing wife/mother etc., and depleted your bone banks, it's time to repay.	Become the remote control queen, whether it's the AC/TV/MiL/ husband/ children. Switch them off when they irritate you.	Menopause is not a deadline that you have to meet before forty, fifty or sixty. It will happen naturally, so don't waste energy by waiting for it anxiously.
If your body is demanding 2 rotis instead of the usual 1 roti — give it, absolutely. The only thing that will make you fat is food obsession not food itself.	Water exercises or swimming is an excellent option. It keeps the hot flushes at bay and improves the tone of your muscles.	Spend a few minutes in silence before going to sleep.	It's not uncommon to feel a void during this hormonally vulnerable time, but it would be silly to fill it up with food.
Your protein requirements go up dramatically, so supplement your diet with whey protein.	Joining a group exercise class where none of your usual acquaintances come is a great way of learning and interacting with new forms of workouts and people. It gets you out of the rut.	Choose sheets, clothes etc. to ensure that all of it makes it easier for your skin to breathe.	Allow unadulterated and free-flow of your emotions, it's high time that you take notice of the 'real' you.
Calcium now becomes a non-negotiable part of your life — calcium citrate at bedtime please.	Trek in the Himalaya, explore new lands and discover the beauty and divinity both outside and inside	Keep a jug of water on your bedside table as you may get dehydrated in the night due to the hormonal shifts.	Menopause may or may not change relationships with others, but it will change your relationship with yourself (and for the better) forever.
Taking antioxidants with Omega-3, betacarotene, selenium, zinc, chromium works to your advantage as well.		Don't avoid carbs for dinner — it helps you fall into restorative sleep and helps you wake up fresh.	Menopause is a time of reflection, self-discovery and of forging new bonds — mostly with yourself.
Your thyroid will be coping with all the hormonal changes and needs special attention — check the chapter on the thyroid (Chapter 6) ☺		The better you sleep, the more stable your moods and energy levels.	

Real life diet analysis
Mrs Khurana is a sixty-five-year-old, pretty pampered ☺ Punjabi lady who lives with her sons, their wives and children.

She has been on a lot of crash diets before, and on all possible diet programmes. She feels she eats little and yet does not lose weight. (Actually, her eating pattern is a classic example of 'fasting and feasting' — not eating for long hours and then eating a big meal.)

She suffers from 'menopausal symptoms' — hot flushes (which is normal) with high blood pressure, knee pain and swelling (actually a consequence of crash diets) — all of which she feels have contributed to her weight gain.

She got married at the age of fourteen (not uncommon) and feels her early marriage has contributed to her weight gain.

As much as she loves her grandchildren, it upset her when they would jokingly ask her which diet she was on now! (She had been on all possible crash diets and would change her diets like clothes ;)). She has the privilege to eat freshly cooked meals every hour and doesn't have any household responsibilities.

Three-day diet recall

Time	Food/Drink	Activity Recall	Workout
Day 1			
5.00 – 5.30 a.m.			Walk
5.45 – 6.30 a.m.			Yoga
6.30 a.m.	Ghiya juice, tulsi leaves and methra		
7.30 a.m.	1 cup tea + 7-8 green almonds + 2 biscuits		
8.00 – 8.45 a.m.		Massage for 45 minutes	
9.00 a.m.	1 glass mango milkshake		

9.30 – 10.00 a.m.		Got ready for a get-together	
11.00 a.m.	Papaya chaat		
11.30 a.m.		Went to market to buy fruits	
12.30 p.m.	Ate lunch out — rajma chawal + raita + bhindi sabzi		
3.00 p.m.	Namkeen seviyan	Moving around in the house	
5.00 p.m.	1 apple	Sat and chatted with daughters-in-law	
6.00 p.m.	Tea + 2 biscuits		
8.00 p.m.	Mango milkshake		
8.30 – 9.00 p.m.		Physiotherapy	
11 p.m.		Slept	
Day 2			
5.00 – 5.30 a.m.			Walk
5.45 – 6.30 a.m.			Yoga
6.30 a.m.	Ghiya juice, tulsi leaves and methra		
7.30 a.m.	1 cup tea + 7-8 green almonds + 2 biscuits		
8.00 – 8.45 a.m.		Massage for 45 minutes	
9.00 a.m.	1 slice of toast with butter + 1 glass fruit juice + papaya		
9.30 a.m.		Went to the temple	
10.00 a.m. – 12.30 p.m.		Went to the market to shop	

11.00 a.m.	Chaas		
1.30 p.m.	Dal + paneer sabzi + salad + raita + 1½ roti	Moved around in the house	
3.00 p.m.	Mango juice		
5.00 p.m.	1 cup tea + 2 biscuits + namkeen seviyan	Chatting with daughters-in-laws	
8.00 p.m.	Maa ki dal + sookha aloo + 1 chapatti + 2-3 pieces mango		
8.30 – 9 p.m.		Physiotherapy	
11.30 p.m.		Went to sleep	
Day 3 (Holiday)			
5.00 – 5.30 a.m.			Walk
5.45 – 6.30 a.m.			Yoga
6.30 a.m.	Ghiya juice, tulsi leaves and methra		
7.30 a.m.	1 cup tea + 7-8 green almonds + 2 biscuits		
8.00 – 8.45 a.m.		Massage for 45 minutes	
9.30 a.m.		Temple	
10.00 a.m.	1 cup tea		
12.30 p.m.	1 glass jal jeera + 1 fruit plate		
1.00 p.m.	3-4 sev puris + 2 bites pav bhaji + dal bati + keer sangi + gatta sabzi + Royal falooda + 2-3 tsp halwa + 2-3 tsp ice cream	Went for a party	
3.30 p.m.		Back home from the party	

4.00 – 6.00 p.m.		Moving around in the house, sitting, chatting	
6.00 p.m.	1 cup tea	Chatting, spending time with family	
8.00 p.m.	1 cup hot milk		
10.30 p.m.		Went to sleep	

Evaluation of the recall

Mrs Khurana believes she puts on weight when she is off any diet programme. She wants to lose her abdominal fat and look slim (again, not uncommon ;)). She didn't want to be off her medication or enjoy good health — she just wanted to 'lose weight' (sounds familiar?). In fact, she believed that taking medication at old age was as common as leaving your mother's house after marriage — something about which you have no choice. She was more concerned about her weight than her health condition and felt that it's normal to gain weight during menopause.

She feels she needs to eat less and so she prefers having a milkshake rather than homemade nashta/dinner and does not eat much through the day. From her recall, we can make out that there are long gaps between her meals and none of her meals are substantial or wholesome.

Menopause is a stage that should be considered a normal part of your lifecycle (just like childhood, adolescence, puberty, adulthood) — only then will your body feel normal and stress-free. Just like menarche marks the beginning of the menstrual cycle, menopause marks the end — so just treat it as an ending (just like every beginning has an end; but just like every ending, it also has a new beginning ☺ — menopause is also a beginning to a new phase in a woman's life.)

All that is needed during this period is love and affection towards your body by eating the right nutrients and nourishing each and every cell of your body (so that even your ovaries feel nourished).

Mrs Khurana just needs to work towards increasing her nutrient stores, improving her bone mineral density, muscle mass and her body composition.

She feels she is eating healthy (she has ghiya juice, tulsi leaves and methra as her first meal, and badam) but she can't do without her morning chai and biscuits. (Remember: herbs like tulsi can't replace your meals — you need to have a good wholesome diet to get the maximum benefit from them.) So her first wholesome meal is her breakfast at 9.00 a.m., when she wakes up at 5.00 a.m. Also she has her badam with chai and biscuits (so zero absorption of nutrients, as sugar interferes with absorption of nutrients), has a big lunch + dinner.

In her attempt to try and eat healthy, she snacks on juices and fruits between her meals. She always focuses on consuming fewer calories rather than more nutrients.

Modifications

First of all, Mrs Khurana needs to eat a meal before her yoga/walk. When we wake up in the morning, our blood glucose levels are slightly low since we have not eaten anything for the last few hours. Eating a fruit would be a good option as this will help optimise her blood glucose levels so she will be more comfortable during her walk.

Mrs Khurana needs to eat well and eat every two hours, rather than have big meals and starve between them. She needs to restrict her tea intake to twice a day and avoid tea + biscuits as her first meal. She can have tea between her meals but not as a meal in itself and needs to completely avoid biscuits (biscuits are loaded with preservatives, especially sodium bicarbonate, which would not only aggravate her already high blood pressure, but also lead to calcium mal-absorption and strip her system off essential nutrients).

She can modify her diet as follows:

Meal 1 (5.45 a.m.) Before walk/yoga: Handful of dry fruits (easy meal, as she didn't want to have a fruit at this time)

Meal 2 (7.30 a.m.) After yoga: Fresh fruit

Meal 3 (8.30 – 8.45 a.m.): Freshly cooked homemade chila/veggie paratha or aloo paratha (Punjabi breakfast)

Meal 4 (11 a.m.): Chaas

Meal 5 (1 p.m.): Roti + sabzi + dal (1 tsp homemade ghee; homemade ghee is good for joints)

Meal 6 (3 p.m.): Roasted channa/peanuts

Meal 7 (5 p.m.): Homemade poha with veggies or fresh fruit milkshake (was very fond of milkshakes and wanted to retain it in her diet)

Meal 8 (7 p.m.): Paneer tikka + green sabzi (I would like her to have roti here, but she isn't ready and actually prefers just a soup, again a low-cal diet fad)

Meal 9 (9 p.m.): 1 cup milk

Mrs Khurana was advised to add supplements for protein (to meet her body's requirements), calcium, vitamins C, E and B-complex, and carotenes to deal with hot flushes, to improve her nutrient balance and to slow down her ageing process (as we age, our body produces a lot of free radicals — the action of which needs to be combated by antioxidants, i.e., vitamins A, C, E).

As Mrs Khurana progressed with the diet, she felt a difference in her energy levels but this was not something she wanted — she just wanted to see a difference on the weighing scale. She was almost upset with her daughter-in-law when she complimented her about looking slimmer! (Though she had lost inches, she had not really dropped kilos as her body was in a state of preserving her lean body mass and bone mineral density, something that Mrs Khurana failed to understand.)

She was resistant to eating often and felt that she wouldn't lose weight this way. I had to eventually succumb to calling it a weight loss diet, only then did she feel that she had lost weight and progressed. So as she 'progressed', her doctor reduced her blood pressure dosage as well, which she was eventually happy about.

Mrs Khurana took at least four-five months to acknowledge the healthy changes taking place in her body — with all the support she needed from her daughters-in-law and grandkids. (On all her earlier diets she had lost weight immediately but lost on her health at the same time. On this one though, she didn't lose weight immediately, but her health did improve.)

She is very happy today and now her grandchildren have stopped joking with her about her moving between diets because she has finally opted for a healthier lifestyle and not a temporary fad diet. She no longer thinks of menopause as a stressful stage in a woman's life — in fact this phase has improved her relationship with her grandkids. ☺

6

Curses We Bring Upon Ourselves

I don't mean 'curses' in a negative way. I mean it in a way where the 'curse' is actually a blessing; maybe in disguise, but a blessing nevertheless. The 'conditions' I've written about below can be seen as an insight that our body is offering into what she is not comfortable with or what she wants changed. It's up to us to take these cues and if needed almost reform or rethink the way we have been sleeping, eating, exercising, relating to ourselves and other people, so not just our bodies but our very personalities learn to bloom. It is our body's way of telling us that it's capable of enjoying better health and energy levels than what it currently is. So don't be foolish enough to blame or get angry with your body — thank her instead.

HYPOTHYROID

What is it? How does it function?
Now before we start talking about the thyroid gland and how/why it malfunctions, this is what you should know:
a)   There isn't enough known about the exact working mechanism of the thyroid.
b)   But there is enough to know that in no way will it interfere with your 'weight loss' plans (so stop blaming your thyroid before reading further).

c)   Nutrition (actually lack of it) plays a huge role in disturbing the thyroid.

d)   Stress (actually our inability to deal with it — blame it on poor eating again) can disturb it too.

e)   Lack of sensible exercise (and no, walked in London/mall-hopped in Dubai/took stairs in office/sat in the sauna don't count as exercise) compounds the problem.

f)   Now I know you will love this one: being a woman does put you at an increased risk of thyroid malfunction.

g)   Pregnancy and menopause put you at a higher risk.

h)   Lack of sleep, recovery and rest irritate the thyroid further.

Okay, enough of the layman stuff. Let's get into the jargon now.

The thyroid gland is shaped like a beautiful butterfly and is in your neck, in front of your wind pipe, just below the 'Adam's apple'. Its function is to produce a group of hormones, collectively called as the 'thyroid hormone'. The thyroid hormone regulates your body's metabolism and the way your body utilises carbs, fat and protein for growth, development and energy in every single cell of the body, not to forget temperature regulation. It also helps release catecholamines like dopamine, the 'feel good' hormone. And it influences every other hormone in the body because, obviously, everything in our body is interlinked. So if one of our hormones doesn't work at its peak efficiency, then all our other hormones, like the growth hormone, insulin, estrogen etc., suffer too. And because they are suffering, it takes a toll on our neurotransmitters and enzymes. And then because our neurotransmitters and enzymes are feeling out of sync, our vitamin and mineral synthesis starts taking a beating. And because the vitamin and mineral synthesis is not up to the mark, our fat metabolism, calcium absorption, sleeping patterns, mood stabilisers, alertness, everything suffers. Get the picture? Our health is like the palace you made with a deck of cards. You remove one card or alter its position, the entire palace looks like it's going to collapse; it may not collapse immediately, but it becomes more vulnerable for sure. Then you do something completely unrelated to the palace, like moving the chair next to the table or bang the door of a room, and *phrrr*, your palace is down.

Chalo, let's get back to the main players in this game. The main thyroid hormones are t4 and t3. Thyroxine or t4 is considered as the precursor (gets converted) to the more active triiodothyronine or t3 and is present in much larger amounts and has a larger half-life than t3 (i.e. it sustains itself longer in the body). Now your thyroid gland is controlled by another gland called the pituitary gland, which is the size of a peanut and is located at the base of the brain. More specifically, the anterior pituitary produces the Thyroid Stimulating Hormone (TSH), which tells the thyroid gland to produce t4 and t3. The pituitary gland gets the signal to produce TSH from another gland called the hypothalamus, which is inside our brain. So the hypothalamus will produce the TSH-releasing hormone (TRH), which will signal to the pituitary to stimulate the thyroid to produce t4, t3 by secreting TSH. Phew!

Let's recap:

TRH →	TSH →	t4 →	t3
Released by hypothalamus, inside the brain	Released by pituitary	The thyroid hormone is secreted, in the presence of iodine + tyrosine, a protein	The active thyroid hormone — triiodothyronine

Now once TSH is released, the thyroid needs iodine and tyrosine to produce t4 and t3. Iodine is a mineral that is very crucial for the body because it's involved in making thyroid hormones, which is central to your body's metabolism. I mean, we all keep talking about sluggish metabolism or have hopes of raising our basal metabolic rate (BMR), but how many of us talk about consuming adequate iodine? Without adequate iodine in your diet, you are fighting a losing battle against fat loss.

Tyrosine, the protein that iodine bonds with to make your thyroid hormone, is a non-essential amino acid whose levels in our body are controlled by an essential amino acid L-phenylalanine. So again, without adequate intake of protein and without the right ratios of essential to non-essential amino acids, the metabolic rate won't rise. Are you getting the story?

Tyrosine along with iodine makes thyroid hormones = normal functioning of thyroid hormones, crucial to optimise metabolism = metabolism that works well = fat that burns well = well, you simply can't afford to be fussy or faddish about your diet.

Okay, okay. It's really not as simple as tyrosine + iodine = thyroid hormone. Many things, enzymes, amino acids, neurotransmitters, vitamins, minerals are involved in the process of bringing iodine and tyrosine together. The chief ones being vitamin B6, vitamin C, manganese, and the enzyme iodine peroxidase (all enzymes are protein based).

So as the thyroid hormones pass through your blood, your brain measures their amount, and if it feels that the amount is low, it will signal the pituitary to secrete a higher amount of TSH. There, you just got declared as having 'hypothyroidism'. No, not by your brain, by your blood test. For the brain is only trying to help you and not label you. A higher amount of TSH is being secreted to help you produce adequate amounts of t4 and therefore t3. It also works the reverse way: when the blood has more than adequate thyroid hormones, the levels of TSH drop.

The family doctor

The good doc is fast disappearing, being replaced by the 'specialist'. You have a stomach ache? Go straight to the gastroenterologist. Got a headache? Straight to the neurologist. Backache? See an orthopaedic. With the 'family doctor' disappearing and losing credentials (in some cases, rightly so), an important link in our health care system is missing. Take the example of high TSH levels (above normal) along with normal t3 and t4 or a high-fasting blood sugar along with normal post-lunch levels. A 'specialist' who spends five minutes (or less) with you in the consulting room is far less likely to make the right diagnosis than a GP who has watched you grow up, knows what your parents' blood pressure/ fasting sugars were like, and has met your husband/children, knows your job profile, working hours, etc. A lot of times, in fact most of the time, you need more than a blood test, X-ray, MRI, etc. to make the right decision about a line of treatment.

Sometimes, plain stress, lack of rest, a bad relationship, frequent flying, the death of a loved one, shifting, change in climate, diet, exercise, can manifest themselves as high TSH or high fasting sugars. What you need then is a professional who is willing to spend time with you understanding the discrepancies in your blood levels and someone who has a fair understanding of your genetic predisposition (beyond the obvious question of 'anybody in family with thyroid/blood pressure/diabetes?) and current changes in lifestyle. A good family doctor fits the bill and can work as a buffer, protecting you from unnecessary medicines and procedures. But then, family doctor, specialist or super specialist, patronising the right and credible doctor is your responsibility. So make sure your doctor (whatever hierarchy or qualification) encourages you to ask questions and answers them patiently in words that you understand. We don't want to pay through our noses for illegible prescriptions written on a shabby piece of paper, but we will pay through our noses, ear, mouth everything to be reassured and well taken care of when sick. Know that it's within your right to be informed about your 'condition'. Know that consent can be obtained and risks of procedures or drugs can be understood only when you are empowered with information, not when you sign on a piece of paper that's called a 'waiver'.

Thyroid and weight loss

Amongst the most frequent questions that I am asked by women who are overweight or those who have 'unsuccessfully' been on many diet plans is, 'Do you think I have a thyroid problem?' Or then there is this final declaration: 'I don't think I can lose weight because I have a thyroid problem'. Or else confessions: 'My doctor/dietician says I won't lose weight because of my thyroid'. And worse: 'I hope I get hyperthyroid so that I can lose weight'!!

So here's what you should really know: if you believe that you have a 'thyroid problem' and therefore must accept a 'weight problem', then you have simply been misled. There is absolutely no reason whatsoever for you to believe that you are doomed or that the body weight won't budge because of a 'thyroid problem' or 'thyroid'. Way too many emails in my inbox have read: 'Hi, your book is great. But I have a thyroid problem so is there some hope for me?' Or: 'Do you think you can still help me?'

Typically, this is what my answer reads like:

Hi,

Thanks for writing in.

Of course the four principles will help you too.

Eating right and working out regularly will help you support your thyroid function and fat metabolism.

Do keep me updated on your progress and stay in touch.

All the best.

Rujuta

You shouldn't feel disheartened about having a 'thyroid'. If you read the first few paragraphs, you will know we all have the gland and should thank it profoundly for all the functions that it carries, not the least of which is fat burning. And calling it a 'thyroid problem', puhleeese! First of all, know that while you were gestating in your mother's womb and were only about three to four weeks old, the thyroid gland was formed under your tongue. Soon it started helping you grow and most importantly started developing your brain, making it sharp, alert, logical, analytical and reasonable. All this work, so that you can function and think 'normally'. The name 'thyroid' is derived from Greek, and it means shield. So the thyroid gland has shielded you from growth and development abnormalities when you were still in your mother's womb, it's been with you since week four. And then by the eighteenth-twentieth week, it also started producing its own t3, t4 so that it could shield your mother from over-activating her thyroid. Now tell me how the ever-giving, nurturing, shielding thyroid must feel when we blame it singularly for our weight gain. We really are so ungrateful! And so stupid too, to feel that all our problems will be resolved only if the thyroid works well.

Our body is interlinked; just one organ/hormone/ muscle/bone/nerve/cell is not causing a problem to our body or life. In fact, our way of life is causing a problem to the entire body and it is simply getting manifested in one of our already overworked body parts. More often than not, our 'problem area' also happens to be the area which has done maximum work for us or has shielded us against all the 'problems' our lifestyle, stress, diet, exercise, relationships, working hours, etc. have caused.

Will it expose me to other curses?

Yes. Leave a thyroid without support (and I mean SUPPORT, not a pill) long enough and it will lead to problems in many other areas. The most susceptible ones are high triglycerides levels (circulating fat which at high levels puts you at risk of developing heart disease), diabetes, sleeplessness, painful periods, constant fatigue, low bone density, low vitamin D levels, and of course weight gain. Sometimes it may even lead to PCOD, high blood pressure … the list really is endless.

And what exposes me to hypothyroidism?

More women than men suffer from hypothyroidism, and the reason is the big hormonal events that we go though in our life, mainly pregnancy and menopause.

During pregnancy, the hormonal balance in our body shifts and our thyroid works very hard to support and provide our foetus with the thyroid hormone; it almost goes into a period of hyperthyroidism. Typically, post pregnancy, if you have taken care to eat right, sleep well and exercise, the thyroid gland will bounce back to normal functioning.

But of course that's easier said than done. Newborn babies barely sleep through nights, so for a mother to sleep well is almost impossible. Post pregnancy, most young mothers are in a state of confusion about what is really good for them. She has to listen to what her mother says, mother-in-law says, the latest women's magazine says or some Pinky aunty's neighbour's daughter says, so to end the confusion she resorts to finishing that ice cream tub in the freezer. And work out? Well, one is so tired changing nappies and feeding, that workouts and gyms seem to exist on some other planet. All in all, in this situation, it's difficult to support the thyroid, but with a little awareness and planning we can do it. The hormonal shift during pregnancy and the shift in lifestyle post pregnancy make the thyroid susceptible to hypothyroidism. So plan pregnancies in advance by eating right at least a year in advance and create avenues for rest and recovery post pregnancy.

Menopause is another time when there is a huge shift in the hormonal environment. It's again a period of confusion about what exactly to expect, and we are often told that a bit of weight gain is inevitable around this phase. False again. Hormonally you are going through a phase called 'estrogen dominance', which means normal levels of estrogen and lower levels of progesterone. This does block your thyroid production a bit and there is always a chance that you may develop 'hypothyroid symptoms', though there may be no case for hypothyroidism as per blood reports. By symptoms, I mean weakness, fatigue, irritability, poor complexion, hair loss, weight gain, bloating, etc. Then of course there are lifestyle and social issues. Most women haven't learnt to speak their mind or haven't learnt to take a break. Working without a break for years together and learning to live with stress puts your thyroid at further risk. Add to that teenage children and indifferent, or worse, demanding partners, and you are clearly overworking the thyroid. So again, with menopause, one needs to equip oneself to cope with both the hormonal as well as lifestyle changes.

Trying too many diets, going to every weight-loss farm, overdoing exercise, being constantly in a state of flux — thin for two months and fat for five months — being on calorie-restricted food, taking 'fat burners' to lose weight and generally pushing yourself to do a lot more than what you have the energy for are all fertile grounds for thyroid malfunction.

What can I do about it?
Tons of things. If we understand that our problem (weight gain or weight loss because of a hypo or hyper

thyroid respectively) is not because of the thyroid itself, then there are tons of things that we can or ought to do. Know that hypo or hyper thyroid conditions both overwork the thyroid gland, so look at your body beyond weight loss and don't tell yourself that I'd rather have a hyperthyroid. A malfunctioning or overworked thyroid finds it difficult to carry out all its tasks, and remember, cellular respiration or uptake of oxygen by your cells is one of them. So work at supporting your thyroid in every possible way. I have listed out the main strategies below. Whether you are hypo or hyper, the points below will help because they are aimed at supporting the thyroid function at peak efficiency so that you get to your optimum body composition and body weight.

Nutrition strategies

- First things first, improve intake of iodine. Before the government decided to iodise our salt, we (Indians) had a lot of cases of goitre. In fact, those of you who are thirty and older will remember seeing women, mostly rural, with huge necks — they almost looked like there was a ball in their necks. That was an iodine deficiency, goitre, another form of thyroid malfunction. It's not so common now, thanks to iodised salt. But it's not just iodised salt that has iodine; a lot of our natural foods that we avoid eating because we think we are fat are actually rich in iodine. Tragic isn't it? Isn't it time we think of our food in terms of the nutrients they provide, and not calories? Or would we rather be on thyroid replacement therapy (fancy name for popping t4 thyroxine/altroxine/thyronom and the like), which eventually teaches our thyroid to not produce its own t4? So come on, let's consume all the nutrients that we need to support a healthy thyroid function, and even if we are taking the morning thyroid pill, let's work at reducing the dosage and finally going drug-free.

- Some iodine-rich foods that we avoid when we go on a 'diet' are bananas, carrots, strawberries, milk and whole grains. I think you can understand why I put bananas, carrots, strawberries and milk in the list of foods we avoid — clearly because they are 'high calorie' and 'fattening'. Gosh! Besides their numerous nutrients, they've got iodine and can help pump it into your thyroid cells, and of course if you are pregnant, lactating or nearing menopause, you need it more than ever. Our thyroid plays a role in the homeostasis of calcium and glucose (it's involved in calcium absorption and glucose metabolism), which means without adequate iodine supply in your diet, you will even become vulnerable to osteoporosis and diabetes.

- Whole grains, read carbs, which is the other food group that we are asked to restrict, if not avoid, when we are on a 'weight-loss diet', are again an iodine-rich source. So please give up on your salad and soup routines and get back to eating your rice, bhakris, rotis, etc. And yes, please eat them with sabzi, because green leafy vegetables and other seasonal vegetables can provide iodine as well. And don't forget dal, dahi or kadhi as an accompaniment, because you need to complete your amino acid profile; remember tyrosine? And phenylalanine, that essential amino acid, to make tyrosine which you will get only if you have good, complete sources of protein.

- So that brings us to good complete sources of protein: cheese, paneer, whey protein, milk, curd, dals eaten with whole grains and eggs, fresh seafood and chicken if you are a non-vegetarian. Here's something funny. On one of my treks to Sikkim, the guide said to me, 'Toh aap "non-meter" ho.' What? I asked. Non-meter = no meat and meter = meat-eaters, he explained. So depending on whether you are a meter or non-meter, choose your proteins wisely. If you are a non-meter, you may need to use high-quality protein supplements like whey protein. Again, as weight-loss victims, we are asked to avoid eating good protein sources. Cheese and paneer are out for being 'fattening', and even if we are allowed dals, it's only without rice and roti, so the little protein that we do consume is incomplete and therefore useless to the body.

- In fact, while on diets, we are allowed such little food and we are on such restricted calories, that even if our thyroid is functioning perfectly normally, it starts slowing down, trying to match its metabolism to the low-calorie diet. And then of course, if we already have hypothyroidism, the diet further weakens our thyroid action by teaching it to slow down more to match the low-calorie diet.

- All in all, if you have a thyroid 'problem', you will need to eat more and you need to increase your calorie intake by consuming more wholesome meals. Got that? **Reassure and support your thyroid with the essential amino acids, good quality carbs**

(unprocessed), iodine, and start taking vitamins B, C and E supplements. Increased nutrient and therefore calorie intake not just supports the thyroid, but it also reassures and encourages it to improve metabolism to match the increased intake.

- Of course, remember that the nutrient to calorie ratio is at the crux of increasing calorie intake. If you start celebrating after reading 'increase calories' and throw yourself a biscuit (however low calorie), ice cream (however fat free) and chips (whichever grain or 'oil free') party, then your thyroid will ruin your party and vice-versa. All processed foods, no matter how sugar-free or fat-free they claim they may be, are rich in salt. When you eat too much salt, then you upset the fine balance of sodium and potassium in your cells (details in Chapter 7) and make it impossible for your thyroid to absorb the iodine that's being pumped at it (now you know why you only have juices and low-fat biscuits and still feel bloated — disturbed sodium and potassium balance). **So remember, increase calories but not at the cost of increasing salt and processed food.** Just have good old homemade and wholesome food.

Peanuts, gobi, soya

If you've got hypothyroid, you've probably been told that peanuts, gobi and soya are banned for you. Why a blanket ban? Apparently, it's not good for hypothyroid? Really, why? Most people who've authoritatively given you this information won't know why or won't have a very convincing answer. But here's the truth behind the ban. These foods can interfere with iodine absorption, but (and this is a BIG but) only if you consume them raw.

Now your peanuts are roasted, the gobi's been made into a sabzi and soya will be in the form of either milk or tofu (and chunks if you are still stupid enough to believe that they are 'protein rich'. No they're not, soy milk and tofu are far superior protein choices). Cooking these foods reduces the antagonist properties of these foods against iodine absorption. So, please, bindaas khao. I mean, just think about it, if the malice 'they' are spreading against peanuts and gobi (in fact the entire cabbage family — broccoli, cauliflower, green cabbage, red cabbage) was actually true, then what about our 'aloo–gobi population'. All of north India dabbaos gobi in the form of sabzi or gobi paratha and even gobi achar. Is there an epidemic of hypothyroidism from Delhi to Kashmir? Similarly, peanuts or groundnuts will find their way into every dish that's cooked in Konkan all the way down to the coastal belt of Karnataka: are we all suffering from the great thyroid disease? (God! And then what will happen to Lonavala chiki?)

The thyroid can't improve or deteriorate because of one thing that you will do or not do. In fact, biscuits, cakes, chocolates, alcohol are a hundred times worse for the thyroid than gobi, peanuts and soya — but are you ever warned against them? Nope! You are sold expensive 'sugar-free, low-fat' versions of these items. And they don't stop at that, they even tell you, Come on, you can't stop enjoying life, so eat stuff which wreaks havoc on your thyroid and be my client forever, dear.

Please note that peanuts and soy are good sources of protein and essential fatty acids, so don't leave them out of your diet. And the cabbage family can lend support to your efforts to eat right by providing you with good amounts of fibre, vitamin B and the microminerals too. So no blanket bans, please.

Exercise strategies

That working out or exercise is a non-negotiable aspect of life, is an essential agreement between you and me, but why is it absolutely necessary for you to exercise if you are hypothyroid? To lose weight? No. To improve delivery and uptake of oxygen by the cells, which will ultimately lead to fat loss. The state where you get mukti from constantly yo-yoing with your body weight.

- It's very crucial that you don't overdo exercise, though, because a malfunctioning thyroid is already a sign of poor recovery. Eating right, sleeping peacefully and working out in a structured manner will ensure that you reap the benefits of exercise without over-burdening your already tired body.

- Cardio or stamina-building exercises are a must to improve mobility of fatty acids in your system (hypothyroid puts you at risk of increasing circulating fats like triglycerides). **Try and perform cardio exercises that will not stress your weight-bearing joints like knee, ankle, lower back and hips.** Cycling and swimming are superb options that provide a good cardio-respiratory stimuli to the heart and lungs while not stressing your joints, tendons, bones, ligaments.

- The thyroid gland secretes t4, t3 yes, but also produces another hormone called calcitonin. Calcitonin works at putting calcium back into the bones. When the thyroid function slows down, it reduces the action of calcitonin too, putting your joints, tendons, bones, ligaments at risk as well as putting you at risk of developing low vitamin D levels (though this is more common after years of exposure to artificial thyroxine).

- **Spend at least one day a week weight-training**, because when you move around with excess weight, the musculoskeletal system needs some serious strengthening to keep you injury-free. Strong muscles, tendons and ligaments protect your weight-bearing joints and provide stimuli for your bones to store more calcium, thus supporting the action of calcitonin.

- **Yoga learned from an experienced teacher can be of amazing value**. Often my clients tell me that sarvangasana is great for the thyroid. See it's like this: first of all you have to learn to perform the sarvangasana with a certain degree of effortlessness (sthiram, sukham iti asana, said Patanjali; it means for your posture to be called an asana, it needs to be steady and happy). To lift the lower body above your head and to hold it against gravity while balancing your weight on your shoulders is no mean task, and to be able to get there you have to first practice many basic poses or yogasanas like trikonasana, tadasana, etc., which are 'not popular' for the thyroid.

- There is no one pill, no one asana, no one thing that you can do for your thyroid. You must be prepared to work on all common sense approaches to help strengthen your system, even if they are not popular for 'helping/curing' hypothyroid. Asanas learnt under expert guidance work on creating a fine balance in the system and work on every single cell of the body, so if you don't get time through the week, find yourself a weekend class. FYI, Iyengar guruji, the living saint, legend and encyclopaedia on yogasana once famously told his students, 'In my opinion if you learn to do the tadasana (simply standing still) well, then you don't have to spend time practising any other yoga pose.' The point is, it's not about how many exotic or convoluted postures you can get into, it's about mastering the asana, and learning to steady yourself in the most basic of asanas or tasks of life.

The morning thyroid pill and mitahar

What happens to Principle 1, 'Eat within ten minutes of rising', if you have to take your thyroid pill first thing in the morning? Well, tweak that principle and make it forty minutes post taking the thyroid pill. The hormone replacement therapy that you are on (ya, I am talking about the thyroxine [t4] tab that you take) is going to interfere with micro-nutrient absorption, so take your vitamins (the multivitamin or vitamin B tablet) only after two hours of taking the thyroid pill. So all vitamins should be taken after Meal 2.

And what about the thyroid pill and early morning workouts, especially if you are short on time? The forty-sixty minute gap that you are asked to keep between taking the thyroid pill and eating something cuts into your crucial morning hours, especially your workout time. Reaching the gym on an empty stomach is not just a guarantee for poor exercise performance but also injuries like sprains, strains, muscle pulls etc. So then what? Simply, speak to your doctor. Most doctors will be happy to work out an alternate time for you when you are on a relatively empty stomach (because the t4 interferes with nutrient absorption and gets absorbed better when you are on an empty stomach). So you can wake up and eat according to the first principle, hit the gym, work out, have a hearty breakfast and go about your day. Your regular workouts will help your thyroid function better and all that you will need to do is stick to taking the pill at that alternative timing that's been worked out for you. Good deal?

Sleep strategies

Let me say this one more time, **hypothyroid is a sign of poor recovery, so sleeping well and waking up fresh are the cornerstones of supporting the thyroid function.** One of the characteristics of an unsupported hypothyroid is feeling sluggish and sleepy through the day and an inability to sleep peacefully at night. (Remember the example of the lady in Chapter 1, with whom all I felt like doing was letting her sleep? Well she did have hypothyroid, and yes, on our third meeting, I did dim the lights and walked out of my office, and she slept uninterrupted for a full twenty minutes.) We all need a good night's sleep. And we all know how zombie-like we feel and yuck we look on mornings when we have twisted, turned too much in the bed and raided the fridge at night. When we sleep well, both the mind and body get a chance to restore a sense of balance and peace, crucial for every cell, hormone, enzyme, organ, tendon, muscle, bone, joint, nerve, etc. in our bodies.

IGF-I or 'Insulin-like Growth Factor' is another hormone that gets secreted by our body when it falls into restorative sleep. This hormone is responsible for a person's ability to recover and grow and allows our cells to absorb nutrients that they need once they are in the blood stream. So to support the thyroid, we need good levels of IGF-I, a) to allow our thyroid cells to absorb the nutrients it needs, and b) to protect us from developing insulin insensitivity or diabetes.

Sleep is also crucial because hypothyroid is affected by what is now being called as 'adrenal fatigue'. Cortisol, commonly called the 'stress hormone', is secreted when the adrenal gland learns to perpetually stay in the 'flight or fight' mode. Hypothyroidism is eventually a condition caused by either hormonal or lifestyle stress, or a combination of both, so expect your adrenals to feel the fatigue. Create good conditions for sleep, and sleep fearlessly in the afternoons for about thirty minutes.

Also, without good sleep, you get zero results out of exercise. So if you plan to seriously exercise, learn to sleep well first. And eating right is a good place to start. It creates the right environment in the body for a restful and not drugged sleep.

And here's a pointer: if you can, then don't wake yourself up every morning with an irritating alarm; instead allow the body to wake up naturally. It's a sign of a good sleep and excellent recovery.

Relationship strategies

Ah! Yes, they affect our thyroid too, simply because our relationships — or lack of them — affect our overall health. It's important to invest time in cultivating and maintaining meaningful relationships, especially with people that we interact with regularly. Having said that, the most important part of the relationship strategy to reduce the load on an overworked thyroid, is the ability to say 'NO'. Say it with me — N.O., NO! Women who haven't developed the skill to say NO are the ones who usually haven't developed an understanding of what to expect out of themselves. On the one hand, they are expert givers — to children, family, friends, colleagues, domestic staff, etc., everybody's fall-back option. On the other hand, they are always left wanting — of others' understanding that they are too tired right now, or must they just do this on their own? But hey, who the f*&$ is asking us to run ourselves ragged keeping up with demanding relationships — mother-in-law wants to shop/maths homework with daughter/movie with husband/presentation at work/making aachar at mom's/

babysitting friend's kid, etc. In every language, there is a word for NO, just learn to say it. And seriously, get over yourself. Just because you didn't do it doesn't mean things don't or won't get done. They will, give it a try, and in case they really don't get done, you already have the expertise and super speciality skill of getting things back on track, right? I am guessing you have realised by this time that you get no medal, trip to Switzerland, gourmet dinner at doorstep, acknowledgement certificate or much less appreciation for being there for everybody every single time, so learn to be there for yourself once in a while. Say no, learn to excuse yourself from all the assumed tasks and responsibilities and listen to your inner voice.

According to the tantric philosophy (and all the eastern sciences and philosophies), the thyroid is considered the sacred voice and corresponds to the throat chakra. A malfunctioning thyroid usually means that you are so busy with life that you haven't found the time or space to hear yourself. Remember how Nandini (Chapter 1) took calls from her daughter, slogged at work, confirmed a date with her husband — all small things, but having an accumulative effect on her stress and TSH levels, ultimately overworking her thyroid. The fact that we haven't learnt to reassert ourselves or talk about our innermost feelings to people who really matter, also adds to the burden. To support our thyroid, we must learn to speak our mind, tactfully yes, but speak for sure. It's often said that women the world over speak the language of silence, and in that process harm themselves and society at large. A lot of women's rights issues are really all about women keeping silent over concerns that need to be made a big noise about or discussed openly and compassionately at public forums.

Alright, I guess I am digressing but here's the long and short of the relationship strategy: learn to say NO and make time to listen to your inner voice (I mean come on, listening to her inner voice Sonia Gandhi gave up the post of prime minister and made Dr Manmohan Singh prime minister. Worked well for us, right?). Here's an idea, take a break (plan for it in advance, of course) for three-four days every three-four months and spend time chilling. Howzzaat? Say that it's therapy for your thyroid. ☺

The Dalai Lama once tweeted: To know what you have done in the past look at your body, to know what you will do in the future look at your mind. And here's my addition, chote muh badi baat (forgive me Dalai Lamaji) — to look at what you are currently doing, look at your thyroid.

The thyroid pill

So if the problem is not an isolated 'thyroid problem', as we have learnt it never is, just taking a pill is not going to resolve it. In most hypothyroid cases, you will simply be asked to take some form or other of t4, but that hardly ever solves the problem, and that's exactly why you will see other women around you taking the drug forever and ever and still having a 'thyroid problem'. The thyroid is only manifesting the problem, not creating it.

If you are already on the early morning pill, then read the strategies that much more carefully, because you need to support your thyroid function more than ever. And don't live in the hope that popping a pill will help you lose weight or complain that even after taking the thyroid medicine you haven't lost weight. I am guessing you have understood by now that just popping a pill is not going to help; lifestyle changes will.

Patronise doctors who believe strongly in lifestyle changes like eating right, working out regularly, sleeping on time and having meaningful relationships whether at home or work. Also doctors who understand that a lack of these factors exposes you to more conditions than ever, and are willing to actively encourage you to change your lifestyle over simply scribbling prescriptions and at the most saying, 'You must lose weight' or 'Go for a walk' or 'Start exercising', while they are scribbling. Mere lip service to lifestyle changes given without eye contact.

Typically, doctors who invest time in working out, eating right and regularising sleeping hours are the ones who have a strong belief in making lifestyle changes to overcome or control (depending on when you catch it) diseases. They believe in them because they have reaped the benefits themselves and are constantly in touch with friends/ acquaintances/patients who have reaped the many rewards. They are fearless about weaning you off dosages, and are happy to walk you to a drug-free state. They also understand enough about drugs to know that the drug can cause side-effects or conditions as dangerous as the disease itself, if not more. Also work with doctors who invest in updating themselves regularly, at least once a year, or those who take study breaks (it's a sign of a responsible doctor, somebody who is willing to let go off his/her daily [big fat] earning to slog it out in school or courses). The rate at which medical science is progressing, it makes sense to stay in touch with the latest, and now of course medical science, especially allopathy (ayurveda, homeopathy, unani and other traditional medical practices have always believed in it), is waking up to the fact that lifestyle changes are crucial for defeating diseases, or at least to ensure optimum or maximum action of prescription drugs and to reduce their side-effects.

How will I know that I am getting better?

Once you wake up fresh, sleep soundly, feel strong in your bones and joints, see an improvement in your stamina and your skin feels better, you should know that the thyroid is feeling supported and will bounce back to peak efficiency functioning. You simply must keep at practising lifestyle changes day in and day out. An improvement in overall health is often associated with an improvement in body composition (more weight of muscle and bone, less weight of fat tissue) and does eventually lead to weight loss. But the reverse — lose weight and you will feel better — is not true. Everything depends on what you lost — bone, muscle or fat. And also what you gained.

Real life diet analysis

Sneha Kulkarni is a sixty-six-year-old TV artiste and a homemaker. She has been suffering from thyroid, diabetes and high blood pressure for the past three-four years. She also has knee pain and digestion problems (stomach gets bloated and has constipation).

She has long days and is constantly busy with household responsibilities, her own work and taking care of her seventy-five-year-old ailing husband.

In her attempt to portray herself as the 'ideal' wife, she has compromised on many things, including her style of cooking and eating (basically given up her favourite foods). She has adapted to her husband's taste in food (they are from different regions and had different styles of food preparation). In fact, she thinks her cooking style, which uses peanuts and coconut, is tasty but unhealthy.

She is concerned about her health and therefore tries to eat 'healthy' (Herbalife milkshakes, Splenda instead of sugar, was her concept of healthy) and has also been to various dieticians in the past. She has gone for days surviving on veggie juices, salads, black tea and pani puri water (this logic beats me)!

Sneha had a lot of responsibilities including work and an ailing husband, and the additional stress of crash dieting amidst all this only led her to a state of depression.

But Sneha was brave enough to opt for immediate treatment to help her out of that miserable state.

Three-day diet recall

Time	Food/Drink	Activity Recall	Workout
Day 1			
5.30 a.m.		Woke up	
5.50 a.m.		Got ready for Hasya club	
5.50 a.m.	1 pear		
6.20 a.m.		Drove 1 km to Hasya club	
6.30 – 7.30 a.m.		Yoga	Pranayam and Hasya yoga
7.45 a.m.	1 peda (clubs are full of these)		
7.45 a.m.		Got back home, went up by lift	
8.15 – 8.30 a.m.	2 dosas with chutney + 1 cup tea with Splenda		
8.30 – 9 a.m.		Read newspaper, made calls	
9 – 9.30 a.m.		Gupshup with my bai	
9.30 a.m.		Bathed	
10.00 a.m.		Went to flat on lower floor to meet husband	
10.15 a.m.	Herbalife milkshake		
10.45 a.m.		Was driven to dentist for treatment of abscess and to fix canine	
12.15 p.m.		Returned home	
12.30 p.m.	Had 2 glasses of water		
1.20 p.m.	¾ bhakri, 2 tsp pithale, 1 serving spoon cooked rice, 1 katori mango pickle		

Time	Food	Activity	Exercise
3.30 p.m.	1 cup tea + 2 pieces chakli + 2 glasses water		
5.00 p.m.	1 mango (small)		
7.35 p.m.	1 glass milkshake (Herbalife)		
7 – 9 p.m.		Watched TV	
9 p.m.	1 mid-sized bowl oats khichdi + 1 katori moong dal varan + mango pickle + ½ katori matar usal + 1 tbsp pithale + 2 tbsp kakdi raita		
9.30 – 10.15 p.m.		Cleared table and washed dishes	
10.15 p.m.		Went to bed	
Day 2			
5.30 a.m.		Woke up	
5.45 a.m.	1 pear		
5.45 – 6.15 a.m.		Got ready for Hasya club	
6.15 a.m.		Drove 1 km to the club	
6.20 – 7.30 a.m.			Practised yoga
7.30 – 8.10 a.m.		Gupshup	
8.15 a.m.		Drove back home	
8.20 – 8.30 a.m.	Two slices bread with 1 cheese slice toasted + 1 cup tea with Splenda		
8.30 – 9.00 a.m.		Made and received phone calls	
9.15 a.m.		Bathed	
9.30 – 9.45 a.m.		Gupshup with my bai	
9.45 – 10.15 a.m.		Internet banking	

10.15 a.m.		Downstairs to meet husband	
10.15 – 11.15 a.m.	1 cup coffee + ½ toast	Gupshup with my husband	
11.15 – 11.25 a.m.		Put room in order	
11.25 a.m. – 1 p.m.		Discussed a teaching assignment with friends	
1.15 – 1.35 p.m.	2 polis + 1 katori moong dal waran + matar cauliflower bhaji +		
1.40 – 2.15 p.m.		Napped	
2.30 p.m.	½ glass Herbalife milkshake		
2.45 p.m.		Was driven to Mahindra Resorts office	
5.15 p.m.	1 cup tea + Splenda + 2 slices of toast + 2 glasses water		
Till 5.40 p.m.		Reorganised Mahindra file	
5.40 – 6.40 p.m.			Went for a walk
7.15 p.m.	Herbalife milkshake – 1 glass		
7 – 9 p.m.		Watched TV	
9 p.m.	1 bhakri + vagyanchi bhaji – 2 servings + chavli plak bhaji + 1 vati moong dal waran		
9.30 – 10.15 p.m.		Cleared table and washed vessels	
10.15 p.m.		Went to bed	
Day 3 (Holiday)			
6 a.m.		Woke up	

6.30 a.m.	1 apple + 1 glass water		
7.30 a.m.		Bathed and got ready for a function	
8.30 a.m.	Tea + sugar + 2 slices mava cake		
9.30 a.m.	4 idlis + chutney + 1 serving rava sheera		
10.15 a.m.		Took a small walk and participated in the thread ceremony	
12.00 p.m.	1 cup tea + 1 slice mava cake	Gupshup with relatives till 1.30 p.m.	
1.30 p.m.	Masala bhaat + turaichya dal waran + 2 servings mixed veg + beans usal + 2 small glasses matha + ¾ katori basundi		
3 p.m.		Drove down back to Pune (driver)	
4 p.m.	2 cups tea + 2 slices mava cake		
5.30 – 6.30 p.m.			Went for a walk
7 p.m.	1 glass milk		
9 p.m.	1 katori moong + waran + 1 serving palak bhaji + 1½ bhakri		
9.30 – 10 p.m.		Cleared table and washed up dishes	
10.00 p.m.		Went to bed	

Evaluation of the recall

Sneha has been a victim of crash dieting in her hope to lose weight and remain slim (read: not healthy) for life.

She was already suffering from a thyroid malfunction, diabetes, blood pressure, all of which are lifestyle disorders arising due to stress, wrong eating habits, lack of exercise and nutrient deprivation.

Crash diets put the body under tremendous stress. Whenever the body is under stress, it releases stress hormones (cortisol) that in turn lead to a hormonal imbalance in your body and increase your nutrient requirements. Along with the release of stress hormones, the body's lean body mass — muscle mass and bone mineral density — is also compromised on (which in Sneha's case lead to knee and bone problems).

So the crash dieting actually aggravated her health condition instead of resolving it. Because of her thyroid condition, she needed to provide her body with wholesome foods along with regular exercise to improve her hormonal functioning. Instead, she was depriving herself of good healthy food.

Modifications

Sneha simply needed to make the right food choices and eat well-balanced meals and also eat to satisfy her taste buds. She mainly needed to create a stress-free environment in her body so that it would be able to maximise the absorption of nutrients. (Whenever the body is mentally or physically stressed, absorption is very poor.)

She also needed to exercise regularly (weight-training particularly) to improve her lean body mass. Regular exercise helps in reducing stress, improves the immune system function, and also improves metabolism. Thus it will help in improving the thyroid hormone function and the cells also become more sensitised to hormonal action. Weight-training will also improve her bone mineral density as it helps the bones retain calcium.

She also joined a 'Hasya club' where she met like-minded people. They took up breathing and stretching exercises as well in this club, which helped her unwind and relax. (A calm state of mind also helps balance hormones.)

She can modify her diet as follows:

Meal 1 (5.45 a.m.): Banana

Meal 2 (7.30 a.m.): Poha/upma/idli

Meal 3 (9.30 a.m.): Handful of peanuts

Meal 4 (11.30 a.m.): Glass of buttermilk

Meal 5 (12.30 p.m.): Rice + dal + bhaji or khichdi + veg

Meal 6 (2.30 p.m.): 2 egg whites
Meal 7 (4.30 p.m.): Vegetable toast
Meal 8 (6.30 p.m.): Whey protein shake
Meal 9 (8.00 p.m.): Fish/chicken + rice + sabzi

She was also advised to take calcium and vitamin D supplements in order to improve her bone mineral density and thyroid functioning. Vitamin B-complex (B6, B12), Omega-3, selenium, zinc, amino acids (whey protein) were also introduced, which together would contribute to improving thyroid hormone sensitivity and functioning.

Sneha adapted to all these lifestyle changes very comfortably. She also followed her diet to the T, except for a few slip-ups on certain days. She was also regular with her exercise.

She started enjoying her food and because of this her nutrient absorption and assimilation also improved. After forty years of marriage, she started cooking according to her traditional style and genes, bringing back coconut and peanuts as part of her diet. Not only did this satisfy her taste buds, but coconut and peanut — which contain essential fats — actually helped lubricate her bones and joints, which relieved her knee pain.

She was motivated enough to feel responsible for herself and not just for her husband. She had started looking at herself with much more affection and this greatly helped her improve her overall health and understanding towards her body.

As a result of all these changes, she started feeling more energetic, and she was able to take care of her husband without stressing about it. As her well-being improved, her husband's health also started improving ☺.

Within two months of making all these changes, her thyroid hormone functioning had improved. With gradual reduction in the dosage, she has now been completely weaned off the medication.

She has now adapted to these changes as a way of life and feels that she has never before enjoyed such great fitness levels while being on a 'diet'.

PCOD / PCOS

What is it?

Whatever it is, it seems to be spreading like an epidemic and is fast becoming everybody's favourite condition to blame their weight gain on! So before we go further into figuring out whether we should blame weight gain or an inability to lose weight on this 'curse', let's get its name right. PCOD — polycystic ovary (or ovarian) disease and PCOS — polycystic ovary (or ovarian) syndrome are like same-same but different. PCOD means that your ovaries are reeling under pressure and feeling the brunt of the disturbances in your body and generally not functioning at their peak efficiency. PCOS means that these disturbances are now no longer just in the ovaries but are also manifesting in other parts of the body — as acne and body hair to put the mildest first. 'Syndrome' is actually like a set or 'package' of symptoms that you get with the 'curse': irregular periods, obesity, insulin insensitivity, high amounts of 'male hormones', irritability, high blood pressure, difficulty in conceiving, oily skin, thinning hair, to name a few.

Now the main problem with this curse is that it often gets 'diagnosed' and 'treated' only after you have been 'trying' to get pregnant for a while. Typically, women who have been married for a while and are having regular intercourse without contraceptives but failing to conceive will be taken to a doctor and declared to have PCOS. Now because the terms PCOD and PCOS are often used for each other, I will use the term PCOS (because I like how it sounds and hear it the most), but know that whether you have PCOD, PCOS or PCO (the last is characterised by the presence of small cysts around the surface of the ovaries; not all women who have PCO have PCOD/PCOS), everything in here will be helpful for you. In fact, the following information will also be helpful to you if you have a thick endometrium and high prolactin.

Before we delve into the realms of our hormones, there are some things that I would like to put down:

- Our body and mind, more specifically, their well-being (or lack of it) affects our hormones.
- Our hormones, in turn, affect the well-being of our mind and body.
- Since PCOS is a hormonal condition, you are up against a vicious cycle and it is normal to feel frustrated.
- Having said that, being frustrated doesn't help. (It may earn you a label though, 'frustu' or 'full frustu', depending on how generous people around you are.)
- There is a saying, 'Complain or do something about it'. Taking inspiration from it, I've coined my own: **'To break out of a vicious cycle, start working with the known factors to control the unknown.'**
- (Thanks for the applause for my creativity; let's get to the point). Between hormones and the body, we know the body better since we can see, touch, feel it every day.
- So let's start working with our body to influence the 'unknown', i.e. our hormones, to which we have little or almost no direct access (mostly we 'feel' hormones only through changes in our body).

- Nobody knows the exact cause of PCOS; it is largely agreed, though, that dropping body fat (that's exactly what your doctor meant when he/she said 'you need to lose some weight') helps the ovaries function better and therefore overcome PCOS.

- On this premise I shall say (no marks for guessing) that I am sceptical about conventional ways of 'treating' PCOS: contraceptives (Yasmin/Diane and the likes) with or without an anti-diabetic drug (metmorfin/Glucophage etc.) and with or without a diuretic or anti-androgen drugs (Aldactone etc.).

- Overriding the ovaries or trying to bring about a 'hormonal balance' by using golis has many issues, not the least of which is the side effects of these drugs. FYI, in Mumbaiya we say, 'Goli mat de', which means 'Stop fooling around'.

- It also means we are trying to work with the unknown to influence the known.

- The more you try grappling with the unknown, the more lost (and fat) you feel.

- So everything that you will read below is the way to use what is within your control (your body) to influence the unknown, which seems to be going out of your control.

Coming back to where we started, the main 'problem' with PCOS is not the fear that it may prevent you from getting and staying pregnant, but the fact that it's stressing your ovaries and affecting the delicate hormonal balance our body tries to keep, day in and day out, minute by minute. Basically, makes it tiresome for your body to maintain good health and immune functions.

Alright girls, we basically need to support our ovaries, and to be able to support our ovaries we need to know a bit about them.

Where are your ovaries? (Before that, ovary is singular and ovaries is plural and since we have two of them, like eyes and ears, we tend to call them ovaries. And mind you, if you don't mind *them*, well then they start rhyming with worries. Ovaries — worries, ovary — worry. Get it?) So ovaries are in the lower part of our abdomen, in the pelvic region, above our vagina. We go about our lives, doing god knows what, and then we stand in front of the mirror and say, 'Yeh mera lower stomach, yeh jana chahiye,' or 'Everything else is okay but my lower abs are bulging out.' Boss, all that fat is sitting right on top of your ovaries, suffocating them, making it difficult for them to breathe, so please, your kind attention is solicited.

Hormonally vibrant

As women, we are what I call 'hormonally vibrant'. We get easily bored with one kind of hormone dominating our system, and since we believe in democracy and equal opportunity, we allow our ovaries to be influenced by different hormones every few days. They (the hormones) in turn, if we allow them full freedom of expression, help us to keep our ovaries strong, well-nourished, oxygenated and vibrant. Ovaries affect the health of our body, and the health of our body affects the vibrancy of our ovaries. Since we're working on the premise that we can influence our body much more easily than our hormones, we will keep talking about what we need to do with our body to make our ovaries healthy. This rhythmic, rise and fall of hormones, almost like a well-choreographed sequence, which happens in our ovaries, expresses itself as 'periods' or 'chums' or menses in our body. Of course we know that this is not just a four, five or seven-day event. When you watch a one-hour breathtaking choreographed dance on stage, performed effortlessly by nubile dancers, we know that they must have practised, practised, practised for hours, days and who knows even months together to put up this one-hour show.

Similarly, for our periods to come effortlessly (regularly), without cramps, mood-swings, etc. our hormones, like the dancers, must work patiently, dedicatedly and practise their moves to perfection under the guidance of a masterji (choreographer). Let's think of hormones as the dancers, rising and falling, twirling and moving; the ovary as the rehearsal stage; the anterior pituitary (you know her right? read Hypothyroid above?) as the masterji; the hypothalamus (you know her too) as the organiser of the show and the body as the main platform where the grand event called menses will be performed. You're still with me, right? Okay, so let's look at what's happening behind the scenes of this spectacular event called menses or periods:

Main event: Menses Day 0 – Day 5	Estrogen and progesterone levels drop low Hypothalamus secretes GnRH* to stimulate the pituitary Pituitary releases LH** and FSH♦ (typically more FSH than LH) slowly and steadily	LH and FSH start producing several follicles (3–30) in the ovary Follicle is like a swelling around the egg (blister type) Follicles starts producing estrogen

Follicular phase Day 6 – Day 14	The dominant (primary) follicles secrete max estrogen and keep growing bigger Estrogen levels in the blood start rising LH and FSH stay low and steady, supporting the follicle to reach maturity	The uterine lining grows due to estrogen stimulation The cervix lining is thin and watery The dominant follicle is ready with mature egg
Ovulatory phase Day 15 Max chances of fertilisation of egg (chances of fertilisation go up if sperm is already present in the system or reproductive tract)	High estrogen levels signal the brain that it's time for ovulation Hypothalamus secretes massive amounts of GnRH Pituitary responds with LH and FSH surge (more LH than FSH) The mid-cycle LH/FSH peak lasts for about twenty-four hours	The pressure inside the follicle goes up and an enzymatic action breaks open the follicle releasing the mature egg The mature egg travels to the fallopian tubes (can survive max 12 to 24 hours) Remainder of follicle (corpus luteum) stays in the ovary Corpus luteum secretes progesterone and estrogen Uterus lining is at its thickest, full of nutrients and well hydrated, ready to receive the egg Cervix mucus at its thinnest
Luteal phase Day 16 – Day 28	LH and FSH levels drop to low and steady levels Estrogen levels begin to drop but get pushed up by the production of progesterone and estrogen by the corpus luteum	The egg starts moving through the tube aided by hair-like projections Uterine lining stays thick to welcome the egg Progesterone levels thicken the mucus of the cervix to stop entry of sperm or bacteria
If fertilisation occurs, embryo secretes another gonadotropin, HCG••	HCG stimulates corpus luteum to produce estrogen and progesterone	Pregnant, and you skip your period
If there is no fertilisation	The corpus luteum starts shrinking and dying Estrogen and progesterone levels drop	The egg passes out of the uterus. Uterine lining shed Menses starts Take it from the top☺

*Gonadotropin-releasing hormone
**Leutenising hormone
• Follicle stimulating hormone
•• Human chorionic gonadotropin

The story of our ovaries

Okay, I agree it's a bit technical. But here's the story in words:

The show organiser (hypothalamus) thinks boss, ek grand event karna chahiye. She has the money (gonadotropin-releasing hormone, GnRH) but not the skill to teach dancing or to spot talent. So she employs a well-known choreographer (pituitary) for the job. On receiving money (GnRH), pituitary sends her team, two teaching assistants, the hormones FSH and LH, for the job. They start talent-spotting and auditioning a dozen or more dancers (follicles which secrete estrogen).

They start putting the dancers through basic but consistent training and soon enough one of the dancers (dominant follicle) shows maximum receptiveness and potential to become the lead dancer. The lead dancer is now almost ready to show off her moves. All this practice, grooming, training is happening in the ovary, the rehearsal stage or dance studio. *The follicular stage.*

The show organiser is happy with the training and gives out some more money (GnRH) to the pituitary, who in turn puts the lead dancer through rigorous training (mid-cycle LH – FSH surge) and arranges for the grand rehearsal with costumes, make-up etc. all in place (uterus thick to receive the egg). The grand rehearsal is thrown open to an audience too (cervix thins to allow sperms). The lead dancer puts up a great show and loses herself (follicle ruptures and releases the egg) in the performance. *The ovulation phase.*

The organiser is satisfied with the grand rehearsal and keeps the money going steady to pituitary. Pituitary's team also keeps up with regular training of the dancer (corpus luteum) and continues grooming it (producing estrogen and progesterone). *The luteal phase.*

As the main performance approaches, the dance teachers decide to taper down practice and allow the dancers to rest a bit (low levels of estrogen and progesterone).

The dancers put up a great show on the big platform that has been provided. The body experiences a beautiful, peaceful and effortless period. Alright hypothalamus, pituitary, ovary, take a bow. Good job! *Menses.*

Pregnancy is a bit like kahani mein twist. Think of it as if some scout (sperm) attends the grand rehearsal, is smitten by the main dancer who lost herself in the performance (mature egg), and asks the masterji to put her through a further nine-month training to put up an even grander show than what was initially planned. Now, not just the masterji but even the dancer herself can start practising on her own (releases HCG) which helps her growth. Nine months later, the dancer surpasses herself and puts up a brilliant show (baby is born).

The story hopefully makes it easier for us to understand menstruation and how the ovaries work under the influence of our hormones and how the hormones that our ovaries produce influence our menstruation and how that influences our body. The reality is, the enzymes which cause the follicles to rupture are all protein-based, made up of as many as a hundred amino acids. The uterine lining, which gets thicker during the cycle, needs an adequate supply of multiple nutrients — good quality carbs, essential fats, minerals, vitamins, etc. — to welcome the egg. As with all fields, the better the platform you provide, the better the performance gets. It means that more and more talent will mature and be eager to perform. Providing a good platform or body is our responsibility. The body is 'annamayakosha', which means that it's affected by food. So if you are keen on providing a good platform to your dancers and want this delicate balance to not topple, please eat right and stop avoiding nutrients under the pretext of losing weight.

So the story above is that of regular periods. Let me take a bow for my choice of words: *regular*, not *monthly*. Because nature doesn't follow standardisation, it prefers the twenty-eight day period to stay in textbooks (mostly so that we can simplify things), but in reality it may express itself every twenty-five, thirty, who knows, forty days. The phase where it varies the most is the follicular phase, the phase where the teachers are spotting and grooming talent. Typically, the older we get and closer we get to menopause, the shorter it gets (maybe the teachers gain experience in spotting, training dancers). The luteal phase tends to stay close to fourteen days. So every woman has her own unique cycle influenced by her heredity, place of birth, weather, nutrient status, exercise status, state of mind, etc. Also the same woman can have a varied cycle every month in different phases (or even months) of her life. So this, 'Oh, my periods are delayed by two days or one week', is really an insight into how little we understand our ovaries. Of course, if you are not getting your period at all or are getting it three-four times a month, then it's a cause for worry, and you could be experiencing the classical symptom of PCOS called amenorrhea (where periods have stopped altogether) or oligomenorrhea (irregular period), the basis of which is anovulation (opposite of ovulation). It simply means that the dance teachers are grooming and training many dancers (follicles) but not even one of them is growing to full maturity, so you have no lead dancer but a lot of mediocre or average dancers not capable of being the lead (producing an egg). This forms the basis of PCOS — poly (many), cystic (follicles, growing like blisters with fluid inside them), ovarian (inside the ovary) symptom.

As I have already said, nobody knows the exact reason or cause behind this 'lot of average dancers and not even one capable of becoming the lead' issue, but there is a huge link with the lack of a good platform (unhealthy body composition or obesity) to this problem. And again, after a problem has persisted for a long time, you kind of don't know what happened first: mediocrity that led to a bad platform or a bad platform that led to mediocrity. So if high body fat made you susceptible to PCOS or PCOS led to high body fat levels, nobody knows, but we all know for sure that they influence each other. Body fat is hormonally active (it's otherwise a 'nonworking tissue' though), increasing the estrogen in your body and therefore putting other hormones off balance.

Also PCOS can occur if the teachers LH and FSH don't divide work equally between them. In PCOS, the FSH and LH ratios — which are otherwise 1:1 — tend to go for a toss, typically more LH than FSH. More LH means that there could be more than the required production of testosterone (often called the male hormone), which again affects estrogen production. The ovaries produce 'androgens' (group of male hormones) which produce testosterone. So consider androgen as a sidekick to the main dancer. No, I don't mean to run it down, only trying to explain that we need androgens like testosterone, but in the right proportion. I mean, what is Munna bhai without Circuit? But if Circuit's role is increased or decreased dramatically, then there is no fun in watching Munna bhai. Get my point? We need testosterone (to keep bone and muscle density, sex drive, etc.), but in the right proportion. As testosterone and other androgens increase, you see their effects on the 'platform', i.e. body — increase in facial hair, hair on chest, stomach, under the chin, change in body fat distribution (bigger deposits on and above the waist, smaller hips), acne, thinning hair, irritability, sometimes even depression. As the platform gets compromised, so does the teaching (LH and FSH), organiser, the money (GnRH) and talent (estrogen and progesterone). As hormones start spiralling out of balance, you start experiencing tender boobs, high body fat levels, irregular periods, heavy bleeding, insulin insensitivity, acne, hair on face, hair off the scalp, difficulty in conceiving etc. (ya, the package). All in all, full-blown chaos.

What does it expose me to?

Well, Type 2 diabetes for one. Long-term effects include high blood pressure, leading to heart diseases, high body fat taking a toll on bones and joints, depression and, not to forget, difficulty in conceiving. The main issue with this is that there is always a chance that you don't get help till you find it difficult to get pregnant. But again, one must remember that 'getting pregnant' is not the be-all and end-all of a woman's life. Know that periods have to be regular and painless; if that's not the case with you, then you need to support your ovaries better and not silence them with a painkiller. Our 'shyness' and stupidity about discussing and understanding our menses can land us with more than one problem. As for getting pregnant, take heart that you are in India. We have technology and doctors who will even make a dining table deliver if they put their minds to it. So seriously, it's not about whether you will get pregnant, it's about how *effortlessly* you want to get pregnant. I mean think about it, more and more women seem to be suffering from PCOS, but has that brought our population down? No, instead we have them giving birth to twins and triplets.

What exposes me to this curse?

Like all curses, there is a genetic predisposition, which means if it runs in your family, you are likely to have it. Before you blame your family, know that a lot of us have this curse today without any genetic link, suggesting a strong connection to a 'modern' lifestyle instead. Lifestyle issue it surely is; I also suspect it's kind of a social issue. Look at the way our lives have changed. Women have made inroads, and successfully at that, in a 'man's world' — they are executives, managers, heads of businesses, leading teams of men and women to make tons of money, travelling more than ever, etc., so they are going beyond 'traditional' professions of teaching, cooking, designing, etc. (men are making inroads here and successfully). Basically, it's leaving women with very little time and ironically limited resources to eat (and cook) wholesome food, so the consumption of processed, quick meals (fast food) is going through the roof. This 'Had coffee for breakfast, grabbed lunch, went crazy with hunger in the evening, only reached home by 9 p.m., so the earliest dinner could be was 9.30 to 10 p.m., had a dessert post dinner' lifestyle is not a good platform to allow our one follicle (come on, it's just one; can't we support that much) to mature. Instead it's a good platform for what is called as 'insulin resistance', which shows a strong link to PCOS. Then there is the fast disappearance of open spaces, limited exercise options, crammed traffic conditions which make walking impossible and turn your fifteen-minute drive to an hour-long one — so, again inactivity and sitting in one place, which only increases your total body fat percentage and makes your weight go up as you go from school to college and from college to work.

According to me, there are 'events' which increase one's susceptibility to PCOS. These are:

- The 10th/12th Std exams where you sit long hours and especially through the nights, where you give up on that one-hour swimming class or whatever little exercise routine you had, to 'study'. You eat chips, sweets, instant noodles, etc. in the night and drink coffee, tea and, of late, 'energy drinks' to study. It's not unusual for girls to gain five to ten kilos in this phase.

- Hostel food, if you went out to study, or the fact that you spend all your pocket money on 'coffee shops and fast food' even if you live at home. Exercise? No. You are in college now, you can't run around in your compound anymore and all gyms/workout places are too far off or too expensive.

- Staying away from home to work. So you may have your own apartment or share it with roomies, but what you don't have is a functional kitchen. So office canteen and instant pizza it is.
- Shaadi-byaah. Now I wrote an entire chapter on this (Chapter 3), so I won't go into details, but yeah, it increases the risk too.

The main challenge here is that we are increasingly living in situations where eating wholesome food in peace and exercising is a distant dream, but where the pressures to look thin are more than ever. Enter crash diets that further cut down on nutrients, instil a fear of food in our minds and deprive nutrients to our already over-worked ovaries. Anorexia, bulimia — basically all eating disorders — lead to amenorrhea or oligomenorrhea, again not good if you want to avoid PCOS.

Eventually you have a brilliant chance to look lean, thin, sexy, whatever your buzzword is, and I am talking of forever, not just for the next big wedding/party/holiday, etc. only if your ovaries are healthy and only if we ovulate regularly.

FYI, women who don't ovulate regularly don't tend to buy sexy, fashionable or nice clothes. They'd rather hide their bodies than celebrate their womanhood. (Nice or sexy doesn't mean short and skimpy; it simply means clothes that make you feel good, attractive.)

Plastic and hormones

Our way of life has changed — we now have more plastic in our kitchen and more pesticides in our food compared to, let's say, just ten years ago. Picture your grandmom's kitchen, your mom's and then yours: how much more plastic is being used now? Now picture size, stress, health issues: you probably score more on every front.

The innumerable pesticides and fertilisers that we are now using is changing our body chemistry like never before. I don't bat an eyelid now when a fourteen-year-old emails me regarding her PCOD, or an eight-year-old turns up with diabetes (Type 2, the adult variety of diabetes). The chemicals in pesticides are making inroads all the way to our ovarian fluid and are busy penetrating deeper into our tissues. The plastic in which you carry your food, reheat, transport vegetables in and stuff take-away in, further brings chemicals into your immediate environment.

There is now a class of chemicals identified as xenoestrogen that are structurally similar to the estrogen that our body makes. The xenoestrogens are environmental polluters (air, food, water) and are a result of increased chemical use in daily life: pesticides, fertilisers, plastic, even fabric softeners, bleaching agents, mosquito and pest repellents, make-up, soaps ... the list is endless. You should worry because 'structurally similar' to our estrogen means that it will take its place in our body. It's like the gold earring you bought where you can fit different coloured drops according to the colour of your dress, or the watch whose strap you can change. Though this means more style in fashion, in our body it spells doom. When the chemical estrogen fits itself into our body, instead of the natural one we produced, it disturbs every other hormone, more specifically our androgens like testosterone. Now you know what that can mean for your ovaries: painful periods, frequent miscarriages, more cysts, high blood pressure, mood swings, more body fat ... the list is endless again.

There is no easy way out. Work actively at reducing your chemical exposure. Do you really need to soften every fabric, switch on the repellent every night, reheat in plastic containers, condition your hair as many times, wash your car with detergent daily? And then do some corrective action: involve yourself in growing at least one tree, reduce garbage in your neighbourhood (to keep pests and mosquitoes out), farm your own food, go make-up free for a day every week and carry food in stainless steel containers (or at least reheat your food in glass: preferably don't reheat at all, just eat and live fresh — top to bottom, all the way).

What can I do about it?

Gosh! Tons and tons of things. Before we go further, know that effortless and regular periods are a natural consequence of optimum body fat, health and fitness levels (it means all hormones, enzymes, neurotransmitters, organs like ovaries, kidneys, liver, etc. are keeping good health). **Feeling comfortable during and before periods is NORMAL. Feeling uncomfortable, irritable, cramping during, before or after periods is ABNORMAL.** It means your health and fitness are in poor shape. It's imperative, and within your reach, to improve your health and fitness levels (not pop pills) to experience an effortless and regular period. The strategies below will help you improve body composition, lower body fat levels and improve insulin sensitivity and work at making the dream of a 'normal, pain-free period' a reality.

Note: Just like around menopause where your periods may naturally get irregular, scanty or heavy, it may also happen at menarche (first period). PCOS is something you may develop at anytime of your 'reproductive age' (menarche to menopause). So make sure you learn to differentiate between the 'naturally' irregular period and the uncomfortable or the unnaturally irregular period. Also, natural or unnatural, these strategies will help.

To begin with, start lowering your body fat levels and make it easier for your ovaries to breathe, please. And no — stop hiding behind the excuse of PCOS/PCOD. 'Lifestyle modification' is the buzzword here. Information is the key. Hopefully you have enough of the first buzzword to write a book now. So let's go to what can we do about it. As always, it's not about knowing, it's about doing.

Alright. Our strategies are based on improving insulin sensitivity (one of the reasons why you may be on 'diabetic medicine' if you have PCOS) and lowering body fat levels, the two main pillars of support for a healthy ovarian function. Easier said than done though, because it's going to take lot of work from your side.

Nutrition strategies

First things first, make time to eat, really. And if you have no time to eat, spare yourself the effort of reading further.

Eating fresh food, wholesome food and eating in peace — you will need to do all these three, together, and at every meal, if you really care about your ovaries. If there is one thing that can really affect your whole life (health, body fat, looks, relationships — just about everything), it's the health of your ovaries. And the most important thing that plays a part in their health is nutrients and nutrient delivery — what you eat and whether it's reaching the ovaries. Simply put, do what you want, pop as many pills as you can lay your hands on, do laser wherever, but if you don't change your current eating (not eating) habits — babe, you're in a soup.

• So avoid soups. **Basically avoid anything that's over-heated**, like an overcooked sabzi or dal that's boiled over and over, or plain reheated or microwaved food. Instead buy your veggies and fruits fresh and don't mash them into a juice or heat them into a soup. Preserve the nutrients by eating fresh.

- Don't go by the diet dictum of avoiding carbs. **With PCOS, you need carbs more than ever, and that too the unprocessed ones** like the humble wheat, rice, jowar, bajra, nachni or ragi, barley, etc. So please eat your roti, rotla, paratha, thalipeeth, thepla, dosa, etc. Whole grain carbs give us the much-needed fibre, which leads to a slow and steady rise of blood sugar (low GI) versus a sharp, fast rise in blood sugar (high GI or processed food). So give up on that 'low calorie sandwich' and eat your roti-sabzi or dal-chawal. Eat wholesome not half-hearted.

- The 'stuff' (hormones, enzymes, etc.) that affects (and gets affected by) our ovaries is all protein based, so **eating complete proteins is a must**. Which means that you can't be fussy and eat only salads: you will need to have dals, milk and milk-products, fish, eggs, paneer, cheese, etc. It's best to take it one step at a time. So to simplify things, begin by adding protein to the meal you have just before starting and ending the most active or stressful part of your day. So spice up your toast with an omelette or paratha with paneer for breakfast, and have a sprouts salad or cheese toast for an evening snack.

Seriously, improving protein intake is not half as complicated as it sounds. Simple acts like replacing colas with chaas or lassi will go a long way. Every amino acid (or lack of it) counts.

- **Stay away from everything that says 'fat-free' or 'low-fat' on the shelf.** Cut the fat from that upper abdomen and waist, not from your plate. Essential fatty acids like Omega-3 and Omega-6, which you can find in ghee, paneer and oils like groundnut, til, sesame, safflower, sunflower, rice bran, olive, coconut, etc., along with nuts, help decrease the glycemic index of the food. I know this is music to your ears — eating fat will slow down conversion of food to fat.

Snacks that are labelled 'low-fat' (FYI, they even sell low-fat butter) rob your body of essential fats, yes, but they also prevent absorption of fat-soluble vitamins like A, D and E. Now you need vitamin D for good bones and for that 'toned look'. And you need A and E for that fresh, supple skin, or at least to keep the acne from spreading.

And while we're talking about fat, have you heard of alpha lipoic acid (ALA)? Well, it's found in flaxseeds (alsi), walnuts and some green veggies. Now here's how it works — it mimics the action of insulin. So if insulin resistance is coming in the way of your fat loss, then all you need is to up your fat intake from sources that are rich in ALA. Btw, peas are rich in ALA too. With ALA in your diet, your body will actually find the nutritional support to pick up glucose (glucose uptake) and other nutrients from your blood stream.

• **Micro minerals like selenium, zinc and chromium improve our body's insulin sensitivity.** Simply put, it helps our pancreas secrete insulin in proportion to a rise in blood sugar. These are found in whole grains, so seriously, don't get swayed by the low-carb/low-fat diets, because you will only be compromising on essential nutrients that are actually helpful to ward off PCOS.

GTF or glucose tolerance factor (the name is self-explanatory; it's like when you hear 'Bond, James Bond', you know what to expect) is a vitamin-like substance that needs an adequate supply of chromium. Eat too many desserts, mithai, chocolate, sweets, and you compromise on your body's chromium stores. Now 'high insulin' or 'insulin resistance' depends on GTF and chromium is part of the GTF. So without GTF your insulin will not be able to pick up glucose from the cells. Insulin and GTF depend on each other and your metabolism depends on the efficiency of glucose uptake. Get it? No switching to nutrient-deprived cereals or 'enhanced' breads or late-night chocolate attacks. Just stick to the basics: **eat often, and eat often at home**.

• **Fresh curd, paneer, sprouts, idli, dosa (anything that's fermented) is priceless for ovaries because of the abundant supply of vitamin B12** (meats are a good source too). B12 plays a crucial role in iron absorption. Low haemoglobin levels are always a factor with irregular periods, lethargy, high body fat levels. Basically it's not uncommon to develop anaemia when you have irregular periods with heavy bleeding (common with PCOS).

• **Calcium is required 'more than normal'** in case you are experiencing PCOS. The cramps, headaches and general fatigue that you feel during periods or PMS will greatly reduce (and eventually stop) if you keep that supply of dietary calcium high. So move over tea at waking up, and late-night cappuccinos — pass the calcium tablet instead.

All-in-all, be a no-fuss girl and eat good food to help your body feel fresh, light and energetic. The hormones will respond by dancing freely and in perfect harmony.

Exercise strategies

1. The worst thing for irregular periods is irregular workouts. **Regular workouts are the key to regular periods.** A regular period means regular ovulation. Now purely from the point of getting pregnant, if you ovulate around twelve times a year, your chances of getting pregnant are much higher than if you ovulate (or get your periods) say four times a year. And purely from the point of getting thin and lean, regular period = hormonal harmony = calm mind, good bone and muscle density = high BMR = low body fat levels = skinny jeans.

Regular ovulation which results in regular, effortless (without the help of a pill and without pain) period depends a lot on how oxygenated and nourished you keep your ovaries. Both oxygenation and nourishment depend on the blood circulation. Blood circulation depends on intelligent activity — read well-structured workouts.

2. Now it's important to not just structure your workout plan but to structure the 'workout', basically the time for it in your day. Too much? Okay, how about this: even seven days of workouts in a month done regularly over four to five months is much more helpful than twenty-five/thirty days of workouts in one month and then zero days in the next few months. Remember, *regularity* is the key here, and seven is a good number to start with. Then as you are able to stick with the seven days a month routine for three to four months, take it to fourteen days. And

then again give yourself at least three months with the fourteen-day routine before multiplying the seven with three and taking it to twenty-one. **The point is not to be over-enthu, just be REGULAR.**

Oh, and it goes without saying, don't ever drop the number of workouts to lower than seven days a month. Read that again. I'm not saying seven *workouts* a month, I'm saying seven *days* a month. I know a lot of over-enthu people will not read properly and give me seven workouts a month by doing two-three workouts in one day. But by doing that, you are letting go of the all-important aspect of training your body to be regular. Got it?

3. **Weight-training workouts are a must** for two main reasons:

(a) They help strengthen all organs — heart, lungs, pancreas, ovaries and the entire involuntary system (that which is out of our control) ka team. Stronger organs means better efficiency. A stronger pancreas means better response of insulin (I keep coming back to this because PCOS has a strong link to insulin resistance or poor response from insulin) and stable blood sugar levels. Stable blood sugar means a much more intelligent use of fat as a fuel by your body. It also means a calmer, steadier, fresher mind. Wow, I have sold weight-training to myself once again and feel good already!

Stronger ovaries mean much more intelligent production of hormones like progesterone and estrogen — basically a much more harmonious situation for our hormones through the menstrual cycle. Hormones in harmony means less cramps during periods, no bloating or mood swings before periods, regular ovulation and an effortless period. Gosh! Why don't we all just quickly do a set of squats in gratitude to the many under-appreciated benefits of weight-training.

(b) After burn. Do you know what that means? See, we all know that when we go for a run, climb stairs, walk, etc. we burn calories, right? And we also burn calories at a rate higher than our basal or resting metabolic rate during exercise, right? Body fat is a major source of fuel for our resting metabolism, so in order to optimise fat burning, we ought to maximise our BMR or resting metabolic rate (basically optimise or max out fat burning during rest). Now after burn means that your body is burning fat at a rate higher than what it usually burns to keep your BMR going. The good news is that post weight-training, your body experiences an after burn for the next thirty-six to forty-eight hours (depending on the intensity of the workout, so do less time pass in the gym). Do the math: invest forty to sixty minutes in weight-training (burn calories during the workout, obviously) and then burn fat at a higher rate than normal for the next thirty-six to forty-eight hours. More after burn means lower body fat levels, lower body fat levels means less hormonal imbalances as high body fat disturbs the natural hormonal balance of the body, especially that of estrogens.

Okay, I know I said two main reasons, but I want to add one for the road. Weight-training leads to denser bones and stronger muscles — which means that sharp-toned body. Come on, move over bra fat (that which juts out from under the strap) and three-tyre stomach and jelly thighs — bring on that LBD.

Alright, so for best results, get regular with weight training and do it at least twice a week.

4. **Cardio is a great way to burn fat, especially if it's associated with learning new movements or a skill.** So how does a nice dance class or kick-boxing sound? Yes, yes, walking, jogging, swimming, cycling are good options too. But since you are going to be spending time burning calories, it just helps if you learn a new skill while you're at it (optimise time). Learning a new skill or art form learnt means better nerve network per unit of muscle fibre (you know what I mean — it's the right hand can write but your left hand can barely hold the pen straight logic. Typically what gets used is what gets preserved and improved upon by the body). Stronger nerve network leads to better strength in the body and helps improve blood circulation too.

5. Yogasanas are a brilliant way to bring about a balance in our entire system, and this balance easily reflects on our hormonal system too. Specifically, pelvic-opening asanas — those which help build strength and flexibility in our pelvic region — are great for our ovaries, and in fact our entire reproductive system, vagina included. Often, along with PCOS comes the banc of bloating, and what better to cure this than surya namaskars, which don't just help the lymphatic drainage, but stretch, flex and move the spine in its full range of movement to provide an excellent stimulation to all the organs (specifically the pancreas and the ovaries) to function to the best of their abilities. **Surya namaskars, along with pelvic-opening exercises, should**

form the basis of your asana practice, but then again, be disciplined enough to learn all the basic postures and make your asana practice a holistic one by signing up with a sensible, patient and experienced teacher.

Weight-training, cardio with a skill and yogasanas are your options — you get to decide what form of exercise you would like to practise more often. If you are going by the minimum seven-day rule, you can spend two days on each of the forms and repeat your favourite on the extra day.

Sleep strategies

As is the case with workouts, with sleep too regularity is the key. **Sleep at the same time every day and wake up at the same time every day if you are really keen on staying hormonally vibrant.** Irregular bed times and, worse, mails, phone calls, TV before going to sleep, can wreak havoc on your hormones if they are already feeling a bit 'off'. And remember what I told you about IGF-1 and sleep in the Hypothyroid section above? Well, that applies for PCOS too (ya, ya, all hormones in our body are interlinked — if one of them is disturbed or out of balance, then the entire hormonal system is disturbed). IGF-1 and insulin sensitivity is strongly connected or interlinked, so if there's one thing you can't compromise on, it's sleep. Also remember, an effortless period (regular) is not an isolated incident, it is simply a manifestation of regularity in your lifestyle. A restorative and peaceful sleep is also crucial for the absorption of minerals like calcium and iron, both of which run low in case of hormonal imbalances or

PCOS. A regular bedtime hour prepares the body to fall into deep sleep and brings about a calming effect on the body and mind, which leads to a sense of harmony for the hormones. An irregular bedtime has the exact opposite effect on hormones — they feel agitated. Late nights also mean a bloated body and sugar cravings the next morning, and you totally don't want that. And just like workouts, it's not like having those eight hours of sleep once in a while, but the regularity of that eight-hour sleep that matters.

Relationship strategies

Typically, an imbalance in hormones wreak havoc in interpersonal relationships (unstable blood sugars leading to irritability, mood swings and low self-esteem). If you find yourself in a relationship where you are taking on more than your share of responsibilities, trust me, your hormones will protest. PCOS (and high prolactin or endometriosis) is simply one of the ways that your hormones are asking you to balance out or share your burden. PCOS/PCOD is an urban phenomenon and common amongst girls and women who have that spark of brilliance and want more out of life. Very often women feel guilty simply because they are achievers (or competitive) at work or college, and they start by compensating for this by doing more than they should, or even more frequently compromising on more than they should be with their husbands/boyfriends. Reasserting your right to lead a complete life or to be an achiever is a big step forward. It's okay to be smarter than the lot, it's not a crime, chill.

The tantric philosophy talks about balance between Shiva and Shakti or male and female energies or that of yin and yang that flow through our body. The analytical abilities, extrovert nature or action-oriented nature is due to the 'masculine energy'. If a woman is in awe of her abilities to think, rationalise and act, then she super compensates by overworking the 'feminine energy'. Some women (mostly older) do it by overtly complying to the 'ideal woman' image of doing everything at home and spoon-feeding husband, children, in-laws, to the extent where they completely run out of energy (almost depression). Others (mostly younger) do it by trying to suppress their femininity (beauty is a virtue of 'female energy') and by 'being the man', or they try and act harsh and cold (manly) even though they may feel warm and friendly from inside. Under-dressing or dressing in a way that almost reduces their beauty is another form of expressing the need to block out the feminine aspect of energy.

Now the problem is that if you under-work or over-work the feminine aspect, you are bound to land in trouble because it creates an imbalance in the masculine and feminine aspects of energy. So learn to express yourself freely and fearlessly. The more you allow uninterrupted or undisturbed flow of energies, the more likely are you to find a balance not just in your energies, but also in your hormones and life itself.

You've heard of the seven chakras? Swadhisthana is the chakra in your genital area and the reproductive system is said to vibrate here. It is supposed to be the chakra for sex, power, money and to all the worldly pleasures of life. It's also linked strongly to creativity (and therefore pregnancy or ability to reproduce). Being at peace with one's sexuality and understanding yourself sexually is one of the ways of liberating yourself from the whole hormonal imbalance drama. Most city folk are tight at their hip or pelvic joints because they either don't fully understand or have enough of sex, power and money. Once you learn to channelise the pleasure part (sex, power, money) of the chakra, the creativity aspect of the chakra begins to bloom. For creativity to flow uninterruptedly you must find that sense of calm and peace in your mind, body and hormones. Creativity also flows when you spend time with yourself learning or understanding your worldly needs and your spiritual needs. Again, to lead a complete life, you will need to seek and gain that all-important balance between your worldly and spiritual pursuits.

Real life diet analysis

Seema Mishra is a forty-year-old housewife who has just given up her job at a bank after eighteen years.

She suffers from a mild form of Polycystic Ovarian Syndrome, resulting in insulin resistance. She has been taking four tablets of Glucophage (500mg) a day (one each after breakfast, lunch, tea and dinner). Sometimes she takes two after dinner. She also takes four tablets of Aldactone (25mg; two at breakfast and two at dinner).

With the diet she was on, she was restricted from having carbs and advised not to eat roti, rice, potatoes, sweets. She does not like this high-protein, low-carb diet (she does not enjoy eating chicken but did so because she felt she 'needed' to). She finds it very difficult to adhere to this on a day-to-day basis and feels terribly guilty every time she slips up or 'eats like us Indians'.

Three-day diet recall

Time	Food/ Drink	Activity Recall	Workout
Day 1			
4.45 a.m.	2 glasses of water (one after another)	Woke up, went to the washroom, freshened up	
5.15 – 6.00 a.m.			Did pranayam, surya namaskars (10), kapalbhati (600 times), brahmri, Bhastrika
6.30 a.m.	1 bowl of sweet melon		
7.00 a.m.		Dropped my daughter to the bus stop and went to the gym	
7.15 – 8.00 a.m.			Worked out in the gym
8.30 a.m.		Showered and dressed	
8.45 a.m.	1 boiled egg, 1 multigrain high fibre cracker (low carbs), half cup coffee (made with ¼ cup lacto-free milk and ¼ cup water) with sweetener		
9.15 – 11.30 a.m.		Attended a job interview. Drove to venue and back	
11.45 a.m.	1 small bowl of salad with capsicum, cucumber, carrot, moong sprouts and lettuce leaves with 1 tbsp light Italian dressing		
11.45 – 12.30 p.m.		Chatted on the phone with ex-colleagues	
12.30 – 1.00 p.m.	One glass water		Ran on treadmill for half an hour at 5.5 miles an hour
1.30 p.m.		Showered again	

1.45 p.m.	1½ cups rice with sukhi prawns, potatoes and cabbage	Feeling guilty as I want to avoid carbs, but when it's prawns it's gotta be rice! God help me!!	
2.00 – 4.00 p.m.		Watched TV	
4.00 p.m.	Half cup tea made with lacto-free milk with 2 tablets sweetener		
4.00 – 6.00 p.m.		Taught my son	
6.00 p.m.	Half Atkins chocolate protein bar (consisting of 8.5 gms of protein)		
6.15 – 8.30 p.m.		Took my daughter for the Speedo swimming class. Drove approx 12 km one way, waited there and drove back	
8.30 p.m.	Had 1 glass of water followed with 1 flour tortilla (carbs 13 gms) + 1 leg of chicken curry, had 1 tsp of sweet boondi (prasad from temple)		
9.30 p.m.		Went to sleep	
Day 2			
4.45 a.m.	2 glasses of water (one after another)	Woke up	
5.15 – 6.00 a.m.			Did pranayam, surya namaskar (80; 20 slow, 60 fast) and asanas for legs
6.30 a.m.	Bowl of sweet melon		
7.00 a.m.		Dropped my daughter to the bus stop	
7.30 – 8.30 a.m.			Bharat Thakur yoga class
9.00 a.m.		Showered and dressed	

9.30 a.m.	1 whole egg omelette, 1 glass lassi made with full cream, yogurt and sweetener	Picked up my daughter from school and brought her home	
10.00 – 10.30 a.m.		Went to Evision counter (300m walking)	
11.00 – 11.30 a.m.		Went to dentist (drove 2 km and back)	
11.30 a.m.	1 glass of water, 1 small bowl of salad with capsicum, cucumber, moong sprouts and lettuce leaves with 1 tbsp Thousand Island dressing		
11.45 a.m. – 1.30 p.m.		Went to hair salon for hair colour touch up, (drove approx 1 km and back)	
1.45 p.m.	1 glass of water, 1 flour tortilla with a small bowl of lauki kofta curry, 1 small bowl of boondi raita		
2.00 – 4.00 p.m.		Watched TV	
4.00 p.m.	Half cup tea made with lacto-free milk with 2 tablets sweetener		
4.00 – 6.00 p.m.		Taught my son	
6.00 p.m.	Atkins chocolate protein bar (consisting of 17 gms of protein)		
6.15 p.m.		Climbed 3 floors to visit friend in building	
8.30 p.m.	Had 1 glass of water followed with a small bowl of palak paneer	Took daughter for a class	
9.30 p.m.		Went to sleep	

Day 3 (Holiday)			
7. 15 a.m.	2 glasses of water (one after another)	Woke up	
7.45 a.m.	Half cup tea made with lacto-free milk with 2 tablets sweetener		
8.30 a.m.			Went to gym
9.30 a.m.		Showered and dressed	
10.00 a.m.		Took my son for French tuition. Walked 200m and back	
10.30 a.m.	1 whole egg scrambled egg, 4 mushrooms (sautéed in butter, garlic, salt and pepper), 1 chicken sausage boiled and fried), half cup coffee made with lacto-free milk with 2 tablets sweetener		
11.00 a.m.		Went to pick up my son from tuition. Walked 200m and back	
11.30 a.m. – 12.15 p.m.		Took my son for a dance class	
1.00 p.m.	1 glass water, a few pieces of paneer tikka and chicken tikka, salad with capsicum, cucumber, carrot		
2.00 – 5.00 p.m.		Watched movie in a movie hall	
3.00 p.m.	Atkins chocolate protein bar (consisting of 17 gms of protein)		
5.30 p.m.	Had tea and nuts		
6.00 – 7.30 p.m.		Cooked 3 dishes	

8.30 p.m.	Had a few pieces of paneer tikka and chicken tikka kabab, along with 1 Diet Coke		
9.00 – 10.00 p.m.		Watched TV	
10.00 p.m.		Went to sleep	

Evaluation of the recall

Seema is making an effort to eat what she thinks is healthy because she has been advised to do so.

Looking at her recall, you can see that she is doing a lot through the day: exercising, taking care of the kids, driving, cooking. At the same time she is making an effort to stick to her low-carb, high-protein diet. In the process, she is starving herself to an extent.

If, instead of eliminating carbs, she eats complete meals of carbs, protein, fats with the right balance of vitamins, minerals and water, she will feel more satisfied with her meals and her insulin response will improve (poor insulin response is a precursor to PCOS).

When carbohydrates are not adequately present in the diet, then the body starts using protein (and later also fat) as a source of energy and therefore proteins will not be present in sufficient amount to perform their important functions, such as rebuilding damaged tissues, building muscles, transporting nutrients, producing hormones, enzymes, etc.

So being on a low-carb diet is in no way improving her insulin response. In fact, because she eats like this, the cells are always starved as they do not receive the nutrients they need. In the absence of adequate carbs, insulin is unable to do this important job of carrying the nutrients to the cells. Fats and proteins, when combined with the right carbohydrates, slow down the release of blood sugar and improve insulin response.

The good part about this recall is that Seema is very regular with her exercise. This is definitely helping her improve her fitness levels, but she needs to eat more wholesome food through the day so that she gets the maximum benefit from her food and exercise.

Modifications

If Seema is more careful about her food and makes an attempt to eat right (not what she thinks is right, but what is actually right for her body) her insulin response will improve (and therefore the PCOS). She will also lose fat and not go through mood swings (a by-product of PCOS and low-carb diets) like she does right now.

The diet recommended for Seema was as below:

Meal 1 (6.00 a.m., after pranayam): Muesli + milk

Meal 2 (8.00 a.m.): 2 egg whites + whole wheat toast

Meal 3 (10.00 a.m.): Laban/chaas

Meal 4 (12.00 p.m.): Poha/upma/idli-sambhar + chutney (she had been depriving herself of 'good food' and didn't have the time in the morning to cook these as traditional breakfast items. She loved it that her 'off time' from jobs presented her with the opportunity to cook and eat — GUILT-free — and that too when no one was at home, so peacefully!)

Meal 5 (2.00 p.m.): Handful of peanuts

Meal 6 (4.00 p.m.): Cheese

Meal 7 (6.00 p.m.): Roti + green sabzi + dal or kadhi

Meal 8 (8.00 p.m.): Glass of warm milk

Seema adapted to this eating pattern and followed the diet to a T.

Her diet was changed regularly to bring in different food options so as to expose her body to different nutrients. She was also asked to take vitamin B-complex, vitamin C, calcium, flaxseeds, zinc and magnesium supplements, as each of these minerals and vitamins plays a role in regulating hormonal action.

She was very regular and disciplined with her exercise as well. (In fact, she was over-exercising in her bid to lose weight. Over-exercising reduces fat burning and leads to fatigue and further hormonal imbalances.) PCOS has a strong link to stress. So though she had quit her job for the time being, she was 'utilising' her time by over-exercising. Physical stress is as harmful as mental stress. She was advised to work out only once a day, instead of twice.

Six weeks after these changes were made, she completely stopped taking the Aldactone. After eight weeks, she was able to reduce the Glucophage to three tablets a day.

By this time she was already looking more toned, feeling much better in terms of her energy levels, her skin was glowing and her exercise performance had improved.

After another eight weeks, she completely stopped the Glucophage.

After all these changes, Seema feels and looks younger than ever before, her skin is glowing more than it has ever before, and she does not feel fatigued at the end of the day. In fact, she feels much more energetic and her exercise performance has also gotten better.

Her periods are regular, pain-free and actually enjoyable — a sign that insulin resistance and PCOS is now history!

Some dope on medicine

Every drug that has an effect has a side effect. That's a rule nobody can deny. If the pill that you are taking for PCOS/ hypothyroid/diabetes/high blood pressure is 'good' for you, then its goodness is also going to do something not-so-good, in fact bad, for you. Only when the 'bad' or side effect is clearly visible do we sit up and take notice: like a rash post an antibiotic will make you think twice about the antibiotic. You will avoid it as much as you can and take it only when you really need to (when you think the benefits of the antibiotic is worth the inconvenience of the rash).

That's the logic we need to apply before taking drugs to 'treat' our 'condition', even if the side effects are not as visible as the rash on the skin. Most of the drugs disturb your intestines, your inner or intimate skin. The medicines that you may be taking for PCOS lead to mal-absorption of the (any guesses?) all-important vitamin B12. Now B12 is involved in some of the really crucial metabolic processes: it is involved in keeping your heart healthy, making your haemoglobin, utilising your carbs right (keeping your energy levels high), helping your neurotransmitters along with B6 and other B vitamins, etc. Very specifically for PCOS, it is involved in reducing elevated levels of homcysteine (an amino acid found in the blood).

High levels of homocysteine (normal levels are not a problem) are associated with pregnancy complications, chronic fatigue syndrome, high blood pressure, heart diseases, etc. Basically it's an indicator of malfunctioning metabolic processes. If you have PCOS, your homocysteine levels are likely to be high (your requirement of vitamin B including B12 is higher than normal), and with the drugs you take for PCOS, it's at a risk of elevating further (mal-absorption of B12) — keeping you in that loop of 'low energy, mood swings, risk of developing high blood pressure, bloating, pregnancy complications' forever.

The thing to do is to understand all the side effects of the effective drug that you are taking as 'treatment'. Is the benefit worth the risk? Popping a pill without doing your risk-benefit analysis is, well, risky.

Know your medicine. I find a lot of my clients not even knowing what they are taking. Like a fourteen-year-old who was on contraceptives but didn't know that she was on one. She thought of it as just 'medicine'. Of course she felt worse day by day, becoming a 'difficult child' for her mother to handle and having some serious mood swings even in school (mood swings are a well-documented side effect of oral contraceptives). Even her mom didn't associate her 'rude' behaviour with the 'medicine'; basically the whole family was in the dark about their little girl being on contraceptives and thought of her change in behaviour as tantrums of today's generation, exam stress, etc. Then there was this forty-six-year-old client who was put on medication for 'low energy' and it turned out to be anti-depressants. She was clueless that she was on anti-depressants, she just thought it was medicine to feel energetic and wondered why she felt sleepy all day in office. Just because something is given to you as 'medicine' or as something 'good for you' doesn't take away your right to know what that medicine is all about. Knowing and understanding what you are taking and exposing your body to it is completely your responsibility. If the medicine doesn't suit you and you tell your doctor about it, she won't beat you up or think you are rude/disrespectful, etc. She may offer you an alternative or change the line of treatment, but give her the chance to know that it's not working for you.

For how long should you take it. The other thing is going on with a medicine forever. A sixty-six-year-old client of mine was on a strong anti-anxiety medicine. Have you been prescribed this, I asked. Well my doctor had asked me to take it for the first flight I took because I was very nervous. When did you take the flight? When I was forty years old. Wow! Does your doctor know that you are still taking it? Ladies, the doctor was as shocked as I was — this lady was supposed to take the drug for just one week.

DIABETES

What is it?

This is easily the most misunderstood problem that we face. The high blood sugar should be the least of your concern babies, the entire FOCUS needs to shift to the *real* problem — starving cells. Yes, you heard me right. **The problem is not that the blood sugar is high, the problem is that the cells are starving.** They are not getting the nutrients which insulin is supposed to deliver to them.

To understand the role insulin plays in our body may be complicated for the world, but it's easy for us Indians. It's the 'middle-man' and we understand the 'middle-man's' role in our well-being quite well, don't we? On one of our exploratory treks in the Supin Valley (tributary of Tons river in Uttarkhand), I came across a beautiful village, Pithari, with wooden houses and slate roofs. As we walked past their community water tap, our guide, lovingly called 'Swamiji' for his environmental initiatives, started taking pictures of the messy scene. A broken pipe, muck everywhere, it overshadowed the traditional wooden crocodile-faced taps. 'Kiske photo kheech rahe ho?' I mocked Swamiji. 'Kichad ki?' In a matter-of-fact tone he explained that the government had just sanctioned Rs 8 lakh (wow!!) to repair and clean up the area around the community water tap and he intended to take before and after pictures so as to hold the 'middle-man' accountable. Even if 1-2 lakh goes idar-udhar, but up to 6 lakh, a larger chunk, comes to the village, it would help them clean up the mess, repair broken pipes and provide clean water to everyone.

Now think of what we eat as the grant of Rs 8 lakh, our cells as the community water tap which is currently messy but needs just a bit of nourishment to get healthy, and the middle-man, of course, is insulin. It is insulin's responsibility to ensure that all the nutrients you consume get delivered to the cells which need them. And it's your responsibility to ensure that your insulin and glucagon (secreted by the pancreas) do their job well. Glucagon is secreted when there is a fall in blood sugars and insulin is secreted when there is a rise in blood sugars (ideally). The only way to keep your insulin accountable for its activity and for its unlimited power to have access to funds (nutrients) and disburse it (cellular nourishment), is to take active part in the process by following the four strategies outlined below.

Nutrition strategies

- Don't skip carbs for dinner, you need them. Simply get the wholesome ones instead of the processed or fibre-enriched variety. Rice, jowar, bajra, wheat, barley, nachni — whatever's your poison.
- The worst thing for diabetes is really low blood sugar. Yes, that's the reason why you are asked to carry a packet of sugar or chocolate on you at all times. But instead of waiting for that emergency to happen, simply eat often, every two/two-and-a-half hours, and of course plan your meals in advance.
- Selenium, zinc, chromium will help your insulin respond better. So go all out to ensure that your food is growing in soil which is rich and not depleted in these nutrients. Also, consider taking these as supplements (of course if your base diet is in place).

- Without adequate protein, insulin will not function well. It will also not function well without essential fats. So eat more complete meals: khichdi + kadhi + ghee or roti + sabzi + dahi or rice + dal + sabzi, etc.

Zinc and added fibre

We need to look at food in totality and not in parts; a self-help book would say 'focus on the bigger picture'!

Fibre is sold as a messiah for weight loss. So there is actually a large population drinking fibre in the night (alone or with a laxative) before sleeping or drinking it before eating, all in the hope that it will 'throw out' cholesterol, fat, toxins, etc. Sorry, no shortcuts. If you are sleeping too late, eating too fast and working out too little, no amount of fibre enrichment is going to help you. It's only going to make you poorer on your fat-burning abilities.

Here's how. Too much fibre comes in the way of absorbing an important mineral, zinc. Zinc is an integral part of our insulin destructing enzyme (IDE) that works at keeping our insulin in balance. Insulin resistance is the precursor to many hormonal imbalances, including that of PCOS, diabetes or plain weight gain. Without adequate zinc absorption from food, we would be struggling with producing adequate IDE and therefore struggling with keeping our insulin in check. Nerds call it hyper-insulimia.

Another problem is that 'added' fibre subtracts the good bacteria from your intestines and actually flushes it down the drain. No good bacteria = poor digestion = high body fat percentage.

So now? Nothing, just the basics — eat wholesome food and stay simple with food. Don't polish or process foods to the extent that they lose all their fibre and don't mindlessly 'add' fibre to your day either.

PS: Just because you are struggling to lower blood sugars or body weight don't just add bran to roti or switch to 'fibre-enriched' biscuits. Spare a thought for zinc absorption.

Exercise strategies

- Working out has a magical effect (without exaggeration) on the glucose uptake of your body cells. To put it simply, it helps you stabilise blood sugar.
- I know you have been advised 'walking', but I hope you will read all the way up to the Four Strategies chapter to understand why it may not be enough to bring about any change in your insulin response.
- Weight-training is a brilliant exercise if you get yourself the right trainer, but that probably means more money. So make your choice: money to the trainer or money to pharmacist/doctor/hospitals.
- Forward-bending and twisting asanas help strengthen not just the pancreas but the kidney, liver and intestines as well. Of course, since yoga is such a misused term these days, ensure that your yoga teacher understands the importance of yama, niyama (the two steps before asana according to Patanjali's ashtanga yoga or eight-fold path to yoga) and is kind enough to impart it to you. And know that to be able to do your forward bends and twisting well, you will need to learn all the basic postures without losing patience.

Sleep strategies

- If there is a first amongst equals, then for insulin resistance/diabetes it is good, restful sleep.
- Insulin functions well only when you sleep well. The problem is most medicines that you will be put onto after being declared 'diabetic' will interfere with sleep.
- No amount of popping pills, avoiding sweets, walking regularly will help nutrient delivery to cells

or lower blood sugar if your sleep is a compromised experience.

- Fixing a regular bedtime and avoiding any sweet post sunset is the best way to keep your insulin accountable.

Relationship strategies

- The body is dealing with the seemingly paradoxical situation of high blood sugar and cellular starvation. Are your relationships a reflection of that? Are you in relationships where you feel loved and nurtured, or are you simply in potentially nurturing relationships and feeling starved for more? Are your relationships 'perfect' on the surface but depleting in reality?
- Another trend that you need to look for is whether you are somebody who is a quick fixer. Are you the type who will allow things to get piled up and simply do a 'quick fix' when it comes to breaking point, instead of learning to take care of things more often or do things on time?
- Being in relationships that fail to nurture (including the one you share with yourself) and allowing things to pile up before you really 'fix' them only leads to a drain on your energy and recovery systems. Soon you land in a place where you have more 'work and love debt' than you can ever repay, much like the nutrient debt that you are carrying in your body.

Real life diet analysis
Jeeva Chowdhury is a thirty-nine-year-old personal banker and the mother of three boys.
She has lived in Surrey, London for the past ten-fifteen years.

Her work pattern is very stressful as she has to continuously deal with clients and barely gets time to eat. Some times, she has even eaten her meals in the washroom!

She feels very lethargic in the morning when she wakes up and feels dull and tired throughout and at the end of the day. She was diagnosed with diabetes, but chose to adopt a lifestyle modification rather than go on OHDs (oral hypoglycemic drugs).

She also has a history of haemorrhoids and fissures and has been taking laxatives almost twice a day for the past few years.

She doesn't eat freshly prepared meals, cooks only once a day, and eats leftovers from the previous day for lunch.

She is the mother of three boys (a Herculean task in itself) and is constantly on the go, which leaves very little time for her workouts (she barely goes once a month).

Three-day diet recall

Time	Food/Drink	Activity Recall	Workout
Day 1			
6.30 a.m.		Woke up	
6.30 – 7.30 a.m.	1 glass water + fybogel	Showered, got ready and helped my son get ready as well	
7.30 a.m.	136g portion of porridge with soy milk + 2 slices brown bread toast with margarine + 1 glass mango and passion fruit smoothie		
7.45 – 8.30 a.m.		Dropped son to school and headed towards workplace. Parked my car 5 minutes away from work and walked to workplace	
8.30 a.m. – 12.00 p.m.		At work, continuous clients, no time to breathe	

12.00 p.m.	Veg pulao left over from yesterday + raita + ½ grapefruit, 1 pear + ½ packet cheese balls		
12.15 – 3.00 p.m.		At work	
3.00 p.m.	1 Kit Kat (4 fingers) + 1 pack of crisps + 1 cinnamon roll		
3.15 – 5.00 p.m.		At work	
5.15 – 6.15 p.m.		Left office, drove to son's school to pick him up, drove back home.	
6.15 p.m.		Reached home, showered son and put him to bed by 7 p.m.	
7.30 p.m.	Dal dhokli + rice and 3 khichi papad		
7.45 – 8.45 p.m.			Went for a walk
9.45 p.m.	Glass of milk + fybogel and Mil-Par laxative		
10.00 p.m.		Went to sleep	

Day 2

6.30 a.m.		Woke up	
6.30 – 7.30 a.m.	1 glass water + fybogel	Showered, got ready and helped my son get ready as well	
7.30 a.m.	136g portion of porridge with soy milk + 2 slices brown bread toast with margarine + 1 glass mango and passion fruit smoothie		

7.45 – 8.30 a.m.		Dropped son to school and headed towards workplace. Parked my car 5 minutes away from work and walked to workplace	
8.30 a.m. – 12.00 p.m.		At work, continuous clients, no time to breathe	
11 a.m.	A cup of tea		
12.30 p.m.	Dal dhokli + rice and 1 spoon ghee, grapes 10-12 + 1 orange		
12.30 – 3.45 p.m.		At work, stressed with clients	
3.45 p.m.	McDonald's chicken select (3 pieces southern fried chicken + sweet chilly sauce + 1 apple pie)		
3.45 – 5.00 p.m.		At work, stressed with clients	
5.15 – 6.15 p.m.		Left office, drove to son's school to pick him up, drove back home	
6.15 p.m.		Reached home, showered son and put him to bed by 7 p.m.	
7.45 – 8:45 p.m.			Went for a walk
8 p.m.	3 chapattis + palak and brinjal sabzi + khichdi + kadhi	Was not very hungry at 7 p.m. so had dinner at 8 p.m.	
9.45 p.m.	Glass of milk + fybogel and Mil-Par laxative		
10.00 p.m.		Went to sleep	

Day 3 (Holiday)			
10 a.m.		Woke up, but lay in bed till 10.50 a.m., then freshened up	
11.15 a.m.	1 cup tea + 2 slices brown bread toast		
11.30 a.m. – 12.30 p.m.		Made long distance phone calls, got dressed, showered, got my son showered and dressed	
1.00 p.m.	Fybogel	Drove to my brother's place for my niece's 3rd birthday party	
1.30 p.m.	Dhokla + chutney, nachos (few bites), cheese and peanut chaat	Lunch at brother's place	
1.30 – 4.00 p.m.		At brother's place, chatting with family	
4.00 – 5.00 p.m.		Went to a funfair with son	
5.00 p.m.		Drove back home, cooked dinner	
6.00 p.m.	Chicken curry + 2 pita bread, rice + salad + ½ glass Bacardi + coke		
7.30 p.m.	Fybogel		
7.45 – 8.45 p.m.			Went for a walk
9.45 p.m.	Glass of milk + Mil-Par laxative		
10.00 p.m.		Sleep	

Evaluation of the recall

Jeeva believes she has put on weight and is low on energy levels because of her stressful work and wrong eating habits. She has also misunderstood her lack of energy levels and weight gain as peri-menopausal symptoms.

She keeps getting sweet cravings through the day (which is very normal considering her eating pattern, which leads to a sudden spike and then a fall in her blood sugar levels).

Jeeva's eating pattern (long gaps in-between her meals) has actually now been well recognised as one of the major factors leading to insulin resistance. From her recall, we can see that she has big meals at a time and then leaves a very long gap till she has her next meal. This pattern leads to a sudden spike and then a fall in blood sugar levels. When there is a sudden increase in your blood sugar levels, your body secretes insulin (secreted by the beta cells of the pancreas), which lowers your blood sugar levels (obviously) but at the same time also promotes lipogenesis (fat storage). Since Jeeva overloads her system at a time (eats a big meal), the pancreas needs to secrete excess insulin to get her blood sugar levels back to normal. Also, to maintain her blood sugar levels during her fasting state (when the levels fall lower than normal), the pancreas secretes another hormone, glucagon (secreted by the alpha cells of the pancreas). So in the bargain, the body's pancreatic cells get overworked (first secreting excess of insulin and then glucagon) and eventually give in — leading to insulin resistance.

This over-secretion of hormones is actually leading to fat storage around her pancreas (stressed out pancreas = fat storage) which is eventually suffocating her pancreas and reducing its efficiency, further leading to insulin resistance.

Also, as the insulin feels overworked, it will lead to imbalances in the overall hormonal harmony. As we now know, this can create disturbances in almost every aspect of optimum functioning of the body.

Jeeva just needed to eat right and eat at regular intervals, which would not overload her system, more specifically her pancreas, and her body could comfortably produce natural insulin (would not need OHDs or external source of insulin). She mainly needed to nourish her cells, since the main concern with diabetes or insulin resistance is not high blood sugars but deprived and undernourished body cells.

Once her cells received the right nutrients, she would be more receptive to insulin and not have bouts of high/low sugar levels (often misunderstood as 'sweet tooth' or 'sweet cravings') through the day.

So an irregular eating pattern, coupled with high stress levels at work, nutrient-deprived meals (leftovers and junk food), no exercise (or barely any exercise) had exposed Jeeva to a lifestyle disorder — diabetes.

Modifications

Jeeva just needs to eat simple nutrient-dense meals, eat at regular intervals (every two hours), nourish her cells with the right nutrients, exercise regularly and sleep on time (which she was trying to).

She had to mainly improve her insulin sensitivity to every meal she ate and turn off the starvation mode that she was in. Once she makes these changes, she will feel much more energetic, fitter, and calmer and she will have a better insulin response. Regular supply of blood sugar to the brain helps your reasoning ability, ability to cope with stress and to make sensible and logical decisions — a definite requirement in a high-stress job.

Once she has all her nutrients in place, her serotonin response will also improve. (Serotonin is a neurotransmitter in the brain which performs multiple functions, including regulating emotions, mood and creating a sense of calm. Stress, nutrient deficiencies, inadequate sleep and insulin resistance are some of the factors that lower serotonin levels.)

She needed to start with regular workouts, especially weight-training, which will sensitise her cells towards insulin and improve insulin response.

She can modify her diet as follows:

Meal 1 (6.00 a.m.): Fresh seasonal fruit (best way to optimise her blood sugar levels and easy to eat in the morning)

Meal 2 (7.00 – 7.30 a.m.): Muesli + milk or oats + milk (easy to eat, does not require any pre preparation and involves minimal cooking [in the case of oats]; she stays in UK, remember ☺)

Meal 3 (9.30 a.m.): Handful of peanuts (easy to carry to work and can also eat it between client meetings)

Meal 4 (11.30 a.m.): Paneer roti wrap with veggies (easy to carry to work and would require minimal cooking in the morning. She could make the chapattis the previous night. Though not really recommended, it's better than having leftovers from the previous day's meal)

Meal 5 (1.30 p.m.): Bowl of yogurt (carry from home or buy a packaged one)

Meal 6 (3.30 p.m.): Cheese sandwich/toast (can carry cheese and whole wheat bread from home or stock her office with it — cheese every day and whole wheat bread every two-three days)

Meal 7 (5.30 p.m.): Soy milk (stock her office with it and have it while she is on the go, since at this time she would be driving)

Meal 8 (7 – 7.30 p.m.): Roti + sabzi + dal (freshly cooked meal at home)

Jeeva also needs to improve her stores of B-complex vitamins (particularly B6 and B12), Omega-3 fatty acids, vitamin C and antioxidants (with selenium, zinc, chromium) — all of which would help improve her insulin sensitivity and ability to deal with stress.

Eating often will leave her energised and enthusiastic about cooking on reaching home and also less susceptible to (and guilty about) 'losing it' with the boys.

Jeeva modified her eating pattern as given and also started exercising regularly.

Within a week's time, she was feeling much more energetic when she woke up, did not need a laxative any more, didn't feel tired/famished even at the end of the day and was just loving the changes taking place in her body!

She also realised that, over time, she was able to deal with her three boys in a calmer and more composed manner than before. Her sleep quality also improved and she would fall asleep effortlessly once she hit the bed.

She also took a much needed break from work (lowered her stress levels), which was one more feather in her cap! ☺

While she progressed, in no time (three months), she realised that she had actually dropped two sizes, from 18 UK to 14 UK! This gave her a big kick to keep with eating right and now she is following it well and is very disciplined about it. She does have a few slip-ups (since she is a big foodie), but she is always aware of it and makes a diligent effort to come back on track every time she does so.

A summary of other curses and strategies to combat them:

Curses	Nutrition strategies	Exercise strategies	Sleep strategies	Relationship strategies
Constipation	Make ghee an integral part of your diet Supplement diet with vitamin B Avoid laxatives and adding fibre to food	Get more active physically in day-to-day life A morning workout may help you activate and strengthen your intestines	Avoid consuming a laxative before sleeping No tea/coffee post sunset	Learn to let go Holding on to grudges, fears, biases, relationships which no longer work has never worked
High blood pressure	Anything that lasts longer than three hours (long shelf-life) should not be on your plate Strictly no salt or masala on fruits	Resistance (weight) training improves the strength and vascularity of your heart. Just because you are ignorant of this benefit doesn't mean that it doesn't exist Work out at least 5 days a week	Avoid buffets and lavish dinners Eating too much in the night only disturbs the cardio-respiratory system and leads to poor/ disturbed sleep	Dil pe mat leh – make that your mantra Anything that overly stresses you is not worth your time, so stop bending backwards all the time
Arthritis/ osteoporosis/ osteopenia/weak joints	Increase protein in your daily diet to improve bone health Supplement diet with vitamin C and essential fattyacids like Omega-3 Have a handful of nuts every day Don't forget that calcium tablet	Whatever may be the level or degree of your joint or bone deterioration, exercise will help, not harm. Of course, make sure you start at the right intensity and don't over or under do it Water exercises work wonders at providing the right stimuli to your joints without straining the tendons, ligaments around it	All of calcium regeneration happens in the night, so you can't afford to not sleep on time You also can't afford to not wake up around sunrise to allow the body to bathe in the unlimited supply of bone-strengthening vitamin D of the sunrays	As women we are more prone to joint disorders, be it a niggling backache, knee pain or a full blown osteoporosis. We are almost brought up to not be strong, whether it's in our body or in our mind Being able to support ourselves is not a sign of misfortune, it is in fact an essential part of adult life

| Menstrual cramps | Too much of sweets or coffee/tea/cola spell doom for your intracellular environment. Stop now

Drink adequate water and check that your urine is clear in colour, not brown or yellow

Double your calcium supplements a week before your period or the minute you feel you are PMS-ing | Olympic records have been broken and made at every stage of the menstrual cycle — pre, post and during — so please don't use this as an excuse to not exercise

But like on all days, be sensible and smart with your choice of and intensity of exercise

Iyengar yoga has developed a full asana routine which helps you ease the flow, reduce the pain and relax your abdomen. What are you waiting for? | There is no specific sleep strategy for your periods. Just use your common sense

Haan, don't feel embarrassed/ashamed/guilty if you stained the sheets while sleeping. It's perfectly okay. Rin ki safedi, okay? Simply put it in the wash | God! You are not impure by any standard of anybody's imagination or according to any religious text

In fact, menstrual blood is used in certain forms of worship as an offering to god, because it's the purest and most nutrient-rich blood (good enough to nourish a life, remember?)

And medical science now tells us that you have stem cells in the menstrual blood which are potentially life-saving.

Will you please have a good relationship with your period now? |

7

The Four Strategies For Well-Being

I

NUTRITION STRATEGIES

Food sustains the life of living beings. All living beings in the universe require food. Complexion, clarity, good voice, longevity, genius, happiness, satisfaction, nourishment, strength and intellect are all conditioned by food.

–Charak Samhita

I was digging into my bowl of fresh fruit, debating whether the 1600m height at Katrain (near Manali) really qualified as altitude. I had given up after just two kilometres of running along the Beas, had tweeted, 'Running along the Beas — the altitude just killed me and the sheer beauty is putting life back into me', and was mindlessly chewing (yes, guilty) my fruits. An unusually crisp, juicy and refreshingly (almost heady) sweet taste brought my attention back to the act of 'eating'. Hmm ... what fruit is this, I wondered. I have always eaten a wide variety of fruits, and I take pride in my ability to recognise the mildest of flavours, aromas, taste, etc. I mean, I have a sharp tongue, literally and figuratively.

So I called on my memory to match this taste, what this fruit was that I was chewing on. It was familiar and distinct and yet not traceable. My inability to 'know' what I was eating teased my mind. I took another bite, chewed it slowly, closed my eyes, opened my mouth wide on finishing and inhaled through my mouth and now used sight, sound, smell, touch, taste, everything I could, to figure out this fruit. Okay, surely it's something local that I've never eaten in my life, I told myself, and marched towards the kitchen.

'Yeh kaunsa fruit hai?' I asked with great curiosity, holding the mysterious piece of fruit in my hand.

'Yeh?' said Bobby (the guy on morning duty) dismissively. 'Pear.'

What? I have eaten pears all my life. I took a bite again — God! It was indeed pear. And it didn't even taste like one. It tasted magical, almost divine, enticing me to use more than one of my sense organs to unravel it, and teasing my curiosity without once revealing its true identity.

So why hadn't I recognised it? Simple. I had NEVER eaten it at its place of origin! So my memory or recognition of a 'pear' was a compromised experience. And trust me, I have eaten good pears, bought it from the best of markets, bought them fresh, eaten them without cutting them into pieces, relished every bite and generally done all I can to get the most out of my fruit. I had overlooked the most crucial aspect though — the pears I'd eaten had always been off the tree for days, may be weeks before they reached the Vashi market from where they enter other smaller markets of Mumbai. During this long and often tiring, uncomfortable journey, the pear had lost its crisp, fresh taste, the colour of its skin had faded, even become black at a few places because of the friction with other pears. With many of its vitamins, bioflavonoids and micro minerals lost, it didn't taste anything like it really should.

Now imagine having a pear which had literally grown ten meters away from where I'd ended my jog, and add to that the fact that it was living on a tree minutes before its consumption. So as my tongue and all other sense organs revelled in its freshness and magical taste, it blessed my digestive system with its mineral, fibre, vitamin and enzyme-rich presence, raising my blood sugar just enough to motivate my insulin to carry all the goodness to my starving cells. Ah! The feeling, the blessing of eating fresh!

And now to weight loss. Why talk of eating fresh? Simply because the better your nourishment status, the better your digestion; the better the digestion, better the assimilation; better the assimilation (and excretion), better the health; better the health, better the fat-burning mechanism of the body; better the fat-burning mechanism (metabolism) of the body, slimmer the waist.

This really is the mainstay of our first philosophy:

1. Eat local, think global

To think big, to think global, to think beyond your limitations, the body must be well-nourished, the mind must be calm. Well that's possible only if the food is richer calorie to calorie, or in non-layman terms, high nutrient to calorie ratio. So theoretically, if you get a hundred calories per pear in Mumbai and a hundred calories per pear in its place of origin, which pear will give you a slimmer waist? I'll give you a hundred rupees if you get the answer wrong.

Here's a simplified correlation for you: **the longer your food travelled before landing on your plate, the longer your navel will travel away from your spine.** Bole ga toh — big fat stomach, three-tyre system.

Eating local and what is in season helps bring the navel closer to the spine and lifts your butt up as well. Also, what grows around the place you stay is equipped to safeguard you against all the environmental challenges that you face. For example, food that grows around the coastal area in an iodine-rich soil condition (kelp, the sea vegetable, is a great source) helps to keep your thyroid healthy. And please can we treat our bananas, chickoo, seetaphal, jackfruit, grapefruit, oranges, etc. a little better now? Chickoo from Gholvad, santra from Nagpur, walnut from Kashmir, apple from Kinnaur, jackfruit from Konkan, guava from Pune, grapes from Nasik, bananas from Kerala — humble origins, exotic results. Or are we going to wait for the West to go gaga over them before learning to accept that these are good for us (we have done it with yoga, we almost did it with turmeric, basmati and cow urine).

So now what? Don't eat those exotic cranberries, prunes from California, olive oil from Italy, the 'English vegetable' from London, the apple from New Zealand and all the 'rich' stuff? Hello! Have it. I am not on a swadeshi morcha. All that I'm saying is that what grows in California will taste and assimilate better in California.

So eat all the exotic stuff, but not at the cost of not eating what grows locally. So another equation: five days of the week eat local or food that has travelled fewer miles, and on two days you can indulge your 'exotic tooth'.

GI

Heard of 'Geographical Identification'? GI is similar to a trademark or an intellectual property. So now we have proper recognition of Darjeeling tea, Banarasi silk, Tirupati laddoo, Goan feni and soon perhaps Hyderabadi haleem. It's a validation of the fact that tea that grows in Darjeeling is unique in its properties, taste, texture, flavour, aroma (read nutrients, discovered and yet to be discovered), and that this uniqueness brings with it advantages to the gastro-intestinal tract or our digestive system that are unique and desirable. Needless to add, removing the foods from their native location does reduce their properties, even if it means their consumption just outside their geographic territory. Now just because Kerala banana or your gaon ka local fruit hasn't earned a GI yet doesn't make it less important or exotic. So please learn to value its uniqueness.

---

2. Portion size

Eating local and eating in season appeals to our common sense, but how much should we eat? Can I eat all I want just because it's local and rich in nutrients; won't I put on weight if I overdo it? Arrey, I know what you want to hear (read) — NO. You won't gain weight. **Mitahar means eating with all your senses, eating healthy (local) and eating in peace, which will ensure that you eat the right quantity.** The quantity of food you consume should be dictated only by your stomach and not by a dietician (or trainer/doctor/mother/any health professional), the latest fad or much less the fear of getting fat. Our shastras say that the wise man knows when to stop eating and the fool always overeats. Now how do you know if you have overeaten? You know it when you experience discomfort or pain later. This discomfort becomes a part of our life, but instead of learning from our pain (yes, pain is our friend), we strangle it with meds, antacids, 'ayurvedic' pills and all the duniya bhar ka kachara. But do we learn to eat till a point where we feel calm, easy, light? No, we learn to 'deal' with the pain of routinely overeating.

There is a saying: if you don't learn from history, history will repeat itself. So if you don't learn from overeating, overeating will repeat itself. Eventually you will lose confidence in yourself, in your ability to decide what to eat, how much to eat, when to eat (and stop), etc. Enter the weight loss industry — toning table, belts, pills, surgeries, low cal food, pre-packaged meals, gym, trainers, dieticians (ya, it's a multimillion-dollar industry out there). The industry thrives on your feelings of inadequacy: you're not thin enough, fit enough, beautiful enough, flat enough on your stomach, round enough on your breasts, etc. Okay, forget it, I am digressing again, but why did I even digress? Because it's relevant to the 'portion' or size of your meal.

See it's basically like this: overeat and it leads to discomfort and pain, with that comes fear. So you stay away from food or starve after an episode of overeating. Now here's the flipside: the other side of the fear coin is greed, so at the next meal you overeat again. Now you're running up and down the bridge which leads from fear to greed; you overeat, you starve, you feast, you fast, you dabbao, you go into a 'can't even look at food' mode again. I so wish this was a vicious cycle, but it's really a downward spiral — at the very bottom of which is fad diets which enforce starvation-like conditions (I mean, please, if you are so averse to eating, just exchange places with one person from the forty per cent of our population that don't get even two meals a day; then at least you can justify the torture you put your body though every time you 'decide' to 'lose weight'), or putting your body through pills, needles, surgeries and a host of other 'quick and guaranteed' methods. And yes, depression, loss of confidence and the host of obesity-related diseases just come with it; package deal, girls.

The rule of UNO
When you run from one end of the bridge to the other, fear to greed, greed to fear, you feel out of breath, out of shape, and out of your mind! Not surprising, na? So then what? S – I – M – P – L – E, that's what my three-year-old nephew Sunay says every time he finds the right piece in a jigsaw puzzle. The missing piece here is making time to eat in peace. When you eat in peace (not in pieces, with your attention also on work, remote control, phone, god knows millions of other things), then you will hear your stomach talk to you. It speaks in a language each one of us, rich or poor, educated or illiterate, fat or thin, married or unmarried, happy or sad, can understand.

Have you played Uno? If you have, you know the rules — when you have just one card left, you're supposed to say 'Uno', or else you've missed your chance and are forced to pick another card from the pack, and that one card can turn your winning streak into a losing one.

Guess you're getting where this is leading. When there is still a bit of space left in your stomach, it says 'Uno'. If you are alert enough to hear that, you put a full stop to your game of eating. If you didn't hear your stomach say Uno, or you heard and chose to ignore it (or you were just 'busy'), then you pick up another morsel and lose at the game of eating 'right', looking thin, staying fit, healthy, happy, calm. Congratulations. And no amount of 'working out tomorrow' or 'slogging at the treadmill tomorrow' is going to change that — you are doomed to stay trapped on the bridge that leads you from greed to fear. To escape the bridge, simply listen, *listen* to your stomach.

Now the stomach will say 'Uno' at different times during different phases of our growth and menstrual cycle. When it says 'Uno' is also dependent on your stress-levels (mental and physical), the time of day, season, geographical location, company during meals and a host of other factors. Women should never, ever (saying this at the cost of knowing never say never) 'standardise' their meal size. **We are hormonally vibrant, and it's perfectly NORMAL to feel like eating more on some days and less on other days.** The key is to stop at the right time. Oh, btw, even our genes can determine the stomach's capacity.

Overeating disturbs not just our feeling of well-being, sense of calm and pride (yes, people; there is a sense of dignified pride in stopping at 'Uno', trust me), but also the hormonal balance, specifically that of serotonin (now emerging as a strong link to appetite control) and insulin (obvious, isn't it?), our satiety centre and of course our blood circulation (that's why we feel so numbed, all we want to do is sleep). And believe me, as counter-intuitive as it may sound, it's really difficult to overeat. Yes, you heard (read) right, it's DIFFICULT to overeat and EFFORTLESS to eat right. The only reason that we manage to overeat all the time is because, as 'modern' women, we are fast losing our ability to rely on our intuition, much less nurture or value it.

Gut feeling
What is listening to your stomach? A gut instinct? Intuition?

The reason why women have been more spiritual than men since time immemorial is because they are gifted or blessed with the power of intuition. Our ancient scriptures tell all of us to be fearless. You get that — be fearless, listen to your own voice and learn to stop eating at the right point. What do we do instead? Listen to our friends, mother-in-law, well-meaning relatives who goad us into eating more ('one day you can eat more/ek din khane se kuch nahi hota/a little mithai is not going to make you into a hippo/oh come on, be a sport have another one/don't be so stuck-up, etc.'). I have been working since 1999, and I have NEVER met a person who didn't know that she was overeating. I have often been privy to conversations that sound like: 'I knew if I ate another roti then I would be stuffed, but I don't know why, I just did it because I wanted my MiL/people to stop talking about my "diet", and after that I don't know what happened I just had a jalebi and then a malai sandwich — full throttle. Now I feel like shit.'

The next time somebody goads you to eat a little more, ask them if they will share your burden of overeating, of hormones going for a toss, of the brain being drained of blood, of insulin being overworked, of fat cells getting bigger, of feeling fatigued, of your heart rate and breathing rate going up, of organs feeling squeezed under fat cells. If they answer in the positive, then maybe, just maybe you can do it. Remember the story in the *Ramayan*, when Valya is asked by Narada if his parents, wife and children will share his karma of being a robber and killing people? His family refused, and Valya became Valmiki. Apna karma share karne ke liye koi nahi aata hai, boss. So overeat at your own risk and discretion.

Eating small

Probably the most misunderstood concept by all those who want to eat right. Once you start practising the four principles of eating right (see Introduction), your meal size may naturally drop or become smaller as a consequence of eating every two hours. But that's not the agenda, really. The agenda is to stay tuned to your stomach and fearlessly eat what it requires. So on a day when you feel like one roti, eat one; when you feel like five, eat five; when you feel like half, eat half. Just make sure you are not crossing the overeating threshold or disrespecting the 'Uno' signal. **Eating right is not about having a 'small portion', but the *right* portion.** And only you can decide what the right portion is for yourself. This is exactly what I tell my clients — as a nutritionist I will help you with what nutrients you need and at what time (based on diet and activity recall). As a person who wants to stay lean and fit for life, it's *your* job to consume the right quantity — not more, not less. Aim to feel light and energetic post a meal, not stuffed and dull.

The one thing that hurts me a lot is to see how my clients who have been to all the dieticians and diets and weight loss programmes in the world still struggle with their weight (because of the yo–yo effect) and lose faith in their ability to know the right amount to eat. Some of them have even asked me to return their money for refusing to 'fix' their portions. 'I just want to eat exactly what you tell me,' said an exasperated client. 'I want to give getting thin a chance.' Well, you stand a chance to get and stay thin only if you listen to your stomach and not me. If I fix your quantity because you don't want to use your brains (ya, she said; if she had to use her brains in deciding how much to eat, then why pay a dietician), then it's going to be a disaster for both of us. For her, because with me restricting her portion, she can eat 'small' for a while, but what after that? She goes back to eating big because she didn't learn to listen to her stomach. Then she may need another diet/dietician/weight loss programme, so it's a never-ending story. For me it's a failure because she would be a client who gained weight post her diet with me. I rate my programme's success based on what clients learn and how well they learn to listen to their stomach, and not on how much weight they lose.

Appetite

Hunger is a sign of youth and health, loss of appetite, a sign of disease or loss of youth. So nurture your appetite (possible only by eating right) and eating well. Often when I am in the

Himalaya for a yoga course, I am amazed at how our genes too play such a large role in our appetites. Even though we all do the same activity, have the same sleep and wake-up times, I find that my Caucasian friends typically eat much more than I do and are just as strong, lean and fit (if not more) as my Asian friends who eat less than them and a little more than me. So it's really not the quantity, it's about whether you are eating 'right' for your requirements and your ability to digest, assimilate, excrete.

It's time to throw away the math we have been fed: calories in = calories out (no weight gain) / calories in > calories out (weight gain) / calories in < calories out (weight loss). Weight gain, loss, maintenance, whatever you are trying to achieve goes beyond maths. It involves the history of your meal pattern and workout status, geography of the place you are currently in — climate, humidity, etc., the molecular chemistry of how the food you are eating is responding with your enzymes, hormones, etc., and above all, the state of your mind. It may sound like the 'it's complicated' Facebook status, but it's not, it's actually rather simple. The point is to keep your focus on the simplest and most obvious part of the equation: are you hungry? Do you feel like you have a good appetite? If the answer is yes, girl you're on track. You're getting fitter, stronger, leaner (ya, losing weight too), and looking like a million bucks! Just keep feeding that fire in your stomach.

3. Food planning

Failing to plan is planning to fail — whoever said this knew how to get the maximum effect from minimum words. Planning to eat right is a bit like that — learning to get the max out of food with minimum effort and tenshun (that's Marathi for tension). So here's the one strategy that you should learn: always plan today what you will be eating tomorrow.

We are becoming experts at planning backwards: self-help books goad us to plan our funeral first and life later. Now if we were to think of our body as the finished product, then the building material or raw product is what we put in it. I'm sure you all know that the quality of the finished product depends on the quality of the raw material, right? So eating local will help keep the raw material fresh, and eating the right quantity helps us to optimally absorb the freshness and goodness of local produce. Now what about the quality of local produce? That's the point I would like to discuss while talking about food planning. All of us want to look fresh and glowing, and be energetic, thin and toned. For that to be possible, we need to go deeper than the maths of calories and look at how our food is grown and nurtured, along the railway tracks or under the watchful eye of a knowledgeable farmer in an unpolluted village on a fertile land that he tills with care, love and compassion?

Food quality

In India, we've traditionally had the practice of storing a year's stock of grains, pulses, spices and condiments that we regularly use. This activity is usually undertaken during summer when the food is first 'sun dried' to fortify the food and as step one of getting it ready to be stored. It's cleaned meticulously, and the storage area is purified and disinfected using indigenous methods and natural products.

No, I am not telling you this to make you feel guilty or to tell you to do behenji giri; all I'm saying is that women spent a lot of time with their food before it came on their plate. And during this time a lot of quality control measures were undertaken. Typically, they also had a fair idea about which field or place their food came from. This means they were quite in the loop about the soil conditions, farm yield that year, the unseasonal showers, the mode of transport used for their food and probably even names, faces and life histories of the people who actually grew their food. You can compare this to wanting to be in the know of the school (schooling and teachers) that your kids study in. We spend time and diligently mark PTA meetings on our calendars, meet other mothers for coffee/lunch or volunteer to do work in school, all to ensure that the quality of education is up to our expectation and because we believe that being involved in the process helps both us and our children grow. We don't think of this as too difficult/downmarket/cheap/behenji types or only for the poor; rather we practically glorify it and take pride in our involvement. Same reasons to get involved with your food and the whole process.

The point is, if food is just landing on your plate and at the most you know which supermarket you picked it up from, then it's like your kid dropping in at home to say she is going from Class 5 to Class 6. Your involvement is close to zero and therefore your control or ability to tell if any learning actually happened is ZERO. Similarly, your ability to tell if your food is nourishing is close to zero. Little wonder then that you eat and feel tired or feel the need to drink tea/coffee/have a cigarette/small piece of chocolate post your meal. Food fails to nourish or energise you; it's almost depleting your energy levels, in some cases actually making you feel dull and drowsy.

Farmers' markets

This is a concept that's big in the world's biggest and bestest city — New York. It's not a concept, it's actually a huge movement, much like the traditional bazaars that India has always had. The Wednesday bazaar or the Sunday bazaar. In fact, small town and rural India is still blessed with bazaars. I just hope we don't lose this tradition to 'development and progress' and then have NY or the West at large reintroduce it to us in a grand, cool way.

So a weekly bazaar is a fixed day when farmers in the locality come to a fixed place and sell their produce. You get the best of sabzi, fruits, grains, dry fruits and at reasonable prices. Good for all. Also it's a great place to bond, socialise and gossip. It's almost a movement in New York: these weekly markets are held in Madison Park, Union Park, Central Park, and loads of other places in the city. So you will have farmers from upstate and NJ selling their stuff and city folk relishing the experience. They even have the best of chefs in the city volunteer to help the 'green movement' by sharing and teaching the crowds how to cook using fresh ingredients to retain flavours and aromas of the foods, and turning them into yummy, healthy dishes. They hand out flyers teaching buyers how to store the food.

In India we know these things, they are a part of our DNA — and if we don't use them we will lose them.

God! Sorry for making your food sound like a nightmare, **but here's what you can do to ensure that food nourishes and not depletes.** Moving back to your village is not what I am suggesting (though that's not a bad idea either).

- Involve your family and make 'know your kitchen' a non-negotiable family activity.
- Typically, just outside of your city toll naka, you will find farms from where you can buy stuff like dals,

wheat, rice, other coarse grains you like — ragi, jowar, bajra. Middle man out, both you and the farmer will benefit. You know a face you can relate to and can ensure that transport is cleaner and faster too.

- This immediately adds value, goodness and freshness to your food. It's time-consuming, and takes effort and planning, but it is truly a rewarding experience, worth every bit of the trouble.

- If this is not possible, pool your resources with a group of like-minded friends and buy some land and learn to grow your food. Don't worry, human resources are plenty in our country and you will learn the ropes of the trade as you grow. Once you have your people growing your food, all that you will need is a 'farm mother', much like a 'class mother', who volunteers to oversee the work and makes regular visits to the farm and interacts with the 'faculty' or farmers. And farm mother can be of either gender, okay?

If you own a farm already, congrats, you know what I'm talking about.

I am not asking you to store for an entire year, I know we mostly have space for about two to three months. But we can start planning for food like the way we plan for tax, reviewing it every quarter, four times a year. Basically we have to stay much more involved with food than the few minutes it's on our plate so that it actually enriches and nourishes our being. To look fresh, energetic and glowing, you should eat food that's fresh, energetic and glowing.

Btw, look at women in villages, they spend a lot of time with their food right from tilling the land, sowing seeds,

278 cs Rujuta Diwekar

cutting the crop, cleaning it, carrying it home, storing it, cooking, eating and relishing it. Who has a sexier figure, a more erect spine and an ageless face? The rural woman or the urban city chick?

Sansar sansar jasa tave chula vara, adhi hataa la chatke tevha milate bhakara — it's a popular Marathi film song picturised on women grinding grain over two stone wheels as they bend, whirl, push and pull to crush the rough grain into a powder that can then be made into a dough, rolled into a chapatti or a bhakri and then put on a tava over a chula for consumption. So the women sing, oh our life or this sansar or world is like the tava on the earthen chula: you will first burn your fingers before you can eat the bhakri or go through hardships before you can bear the fruit of your effort. So how far are you willing to go to get that fab body? All the way to the fields?

How far will you go?

Here's one of my favourite stories that a client from Surat shared. One of his friends (yup, diamond merchant by profession) owns a farm on which he grows lots of local fruits and vegetables. The vegetables from his farm are especially yummy, and he is really keen that his brother, who lives in Mumbai, not miss out on them. So early every morning (yes, every single day), one of his men goes to the farm, picks up some fresh vegetables, puts them in a basket, goes to Surat station and puts the basket under a seat in one of the super-fast trains. He then sms-es the seat number to the man in Mumbai, someone is sent to pick it up from Mumbai central, it enters bhabi's kitchen, brother's plate and eventually his stomach. Nine times out of ten, he is able to get the vegetable basket, once in a while some passenger on the train gets lucky!

4. Beyond calories

I felt I had walked endlessly by the Pin river after crossing the Bhabha pass at 4900 meters. Tired, dazed and out of breath, I kept moving my legs and finally by evening I'd reached a bridge across which sat the village of Mudh. Anatomically it looks like a vagina, is what I thought to myself. It's a village with pinkish red and white homes fed by streams from two sides and it sits in the V shape in between. Awesome, I thought.

As I negotiated with my lungs and my heart started feeling light and nice, my eyes caught sight of women and children in fields where peas were being grown. The women walked up to the trail (Spitians are super friendly), bringing with them a handful of peas for me. I was more than happy to eat something so I peeled a pod, admiring how refreshingly green the peas and the peel looked (they always look tired, patchy almost greyish in Mumbai markets). I popped the peas in my mouth — Ah, god, sweeter than sugar, I could feel fatigue vanishing from my legs and mind. 'Now eat the peel,' said the lady.

What? I may look like a monkey but I am not one, I wanted to say, but I don't take panga with locals, especially when they are in a group. So I obediently put the peel in my mouth. *Kaaraak*, it broke between my teeth and its juice sprayed across my palette and I heard myself go, Hmmm, wow! (The only expression I'd said aloud since crossing the pass.) The women giggled. You must always eat the peel, the oldest amongst them said. Good for your skin. Wow! I didn't want to tell her what happens to peas back home so I can't follow her advice as much as I believed her and would want to recreate my HMMM experience.

But why am I telling you this? Because food is not about numbers or, more specifically, calories. It's about feelings, emotion, romance, enriching and rewarding and central to human existence. It's high time we think nutrients (and our emotions while eating and the farming community's while growing, not to mention our cook's while cooking) and not calories. So this lamba chauda story is to tell you that every time somebody dismisses peas as a 'high calorie' veggie, I feel heartbroken, or rather, devastated. Peas are rich in potassium (something that could rid you of chronic bloating), vitamins B1, B2, B3 (great for when you feel tired), A, C, K and E, apart from calcium, selenium, iron, and zinc, enzymes, natural sugars, fibres. So much goodness all dismissed because it's 'badnaam' thanks to calories.

Sodium-potassium pump

During my treks with 'Connect with Himalaya', I am often amazed at how GP is much faster and 'luckier' than I am when it comes to spotting wildlife. 'The key is to look at the right places,' he explained when he sensed my envy. What's a 'right place', I asked, irritated. 'Dry streams, the animals often come to dry streams to lick the salt and mineral deposits off the river bed,' he explained. We are all wired to pick up and look for salt, specifically for sodium, because we are supposed to get adequate amounts of potassium from the food we eat. Yes, I am talking about the **sodium-potassium pump**. Potassium is part of what is called as intracellular or inside the cell fluid; sodium is a part of the extracellular fluid or the fluid that is outside the cells. How well our cells absorb nutrients from the blood stream, throw out waste, respond and send nerve impulses, in fact every minute function that our cells carry out depends on whether they have the right amount of sodium outside and potassium inside. Together, the sodium and potassium make the electrochemical impulse, or current-making movement inside and outside the cell, smooth and easy, in fact, possible.

Our diets, which are getting increasingly high in sodium thanks to the consumption of processed foods, fast foods and take-aways, are proving to be a big challenge to our delicately maintained Na–K pump. Add to that the fact that we are getting increasingly less fresh food, farming practices have changed and fertiliser use is higher than ever, all of which depletes the potassium stores in our body. Now when sodium increases and potassium drops, the sodium forces its way inside the cell and from there on starts the slow death of our cells because of impaired absorption of nutrients and inability to throw out waste products. Bloating or swelling is the first visible sign of this disturbed electro-chemical balance. So the next time you call for food from outside, eat too late, open a packet of diet chakli/chips, and on the other hand avoid eating 'fattening' bananas, potatoes, etc., spare a thought for the Na-K pump and the impending slow death of cells.

Nutrients

So this is where you should use buddhi, intuition and intelligence the next time somebody calls our nutrient-rich peas, carrots, potatoes, suran, sweet potato, beetroot, mangoes, rice, seetaphal, banana, chickoo, etc. 'high calorie'. Please dimaag lagao; in Marathi there's a term for this — akal ghan takli ka? (loosely translated to 'have you mortgaged your brains?', used when you can't fathom really, really BASIC ideas).

You know this math? 1g carb = 4 calories, 1g protein – 4 calories, 1g of fat = 9 calories. Now if food, naturally existing in nature, is 'calorie-rich', what does it mean? That it's NUTRIENT-RICH! Oh, I have to stop screaming and stop being rude. So sorry for lacking the tact to say it in a more appropriate manner — but you are saying NO to nutrients. Food that exists in its pure form in nature on trees, grass, shrubs, creepers, etc. as a fruit, vegetable, grain, pulse is not 'fattening'. The calories are coming from the nutrients — carbs, protein, fat (usually a really small contribution) — and we need all these in our body to assimilate all the micro-nutrients like vitamins and minerals. Without adequate nutrients — the whole lot of them: carbs, protein, fat, vitamins, minerals, water, fibre — our body would never be able to enjoy optimum health, fitness or wellness. When a sense of well-being is lacking, you don't *feel* beautiful. Instead, you constantly feel inadequate.

So use your brains: if you're messing around with your fruits, vegetables, grains and processing them to a point where they've lost their nutrients and fibres, like turning them into a pulp, pickle, jam, biscuit, pastry, fruit cake, juice or frying them into chips, then yes, you're adding to the calories and removing nutrients. Avoid this messing with your food in the name of 'convenience', 'handy', 'quick snack', and to avoid calories. Calories are a good thing, trust me. On the one hand you want to look fresh and feel energetic, and on the other you want to avoid calories. **Every time you say no to calories, you say no to energy.** Energy and calories are the exact same thing. If output (body) has to be energetic, then the input (food) has to have calories. Annamaya kosha — the body is made of food. If your food is frozen, preserved, heavy on preservatives, overcooked or stale, what is your body going to look like? Anybody wants to take a wild guess?

Are you avoiding calories? Is this what your diet plan looks like?

Cereal + low fat milk

Juice

Salad with whole wheat toast

Fruit

Dry bhel or mumra

Fibre-added roti and boiled vegetables

God! Your body is going to look like it's in mourning. The cereal is rich in preservatives and sodium and perhaps also emulsifiers and permitted additives; the milk is stripped of its main nutrient, the essential fat; the juice is coloured water, stripped of fibre; the salad's been cut god knows when, and god forbid if you added low-fat dressing to give your body its daily quota of preservatives and salt; the whole wheat loaf has a shelf-life higher than chapatti so you know what *that* means; the fruit, well, what are you thinking? The body needs proper carbs, protein, fat to assimilate anything from the fruit. The dry bhel is an atyachar on your palate so the enzymes won't be interested and optimum digestion itself will not take place. The fibre 'added' to the roti is only going to 'add' to your body's woes of absorbing calcium and iron. Wow! No wonder you don't lose fat on a diet like this (weight you could lose, and with it your charm, energy and sleep).

My name is carb and I am not fattening

Inspired entirely by *My Name is Khan* (and I am not a terrorist). When you take out of a potato, banana, rice, wheat (also seetaphal, chickoo, mango, grapes) what makes them nutritious and energy-giving and turn them into items that are filled with preservatives, additives, permitted colourings, emulsifiers, salts and, worse, the added 'healthy' fibre, calcium, iron, etc., they no longer remain usable for the body.

Just like terror has no colour or religion, junk has no health or nutritional value.

Actually, adding 'health' or 'religion' to junk may sell it better and even find credibility with the gullible, but does it help add to physical, emotional, mental, spiritual well-being? No, it erodes it in a cruel manner, bringing disrepute to the entire 'food group' or 'community', spreads fear and makes our lives dull, limited and boring. Think about how the roti and rice feel when you leave it out of your life, thinking that they are harmful, and choose to eat only salad or soup or sabzi + dal? Devastated, misunderstood and let down, you bet.

So when you remove fibre, niacin and vitamin B, zinc, selenium and a host of other vitamins, minerals and enzymes from carbs, it no longer remains a carb, it simply turns to junk. Is junk fattening? Yes. Can you turn carb to junk? Yes, by removing all that makes it a carb. You could apply the same process to protein, fat, water and turn them to junk too. (Water to cola, meat to sausage, white butter to yellow butter or margarine). Just because they do it primarily with carbs, it hasn't earned them that label yet. And avoiding carbs is leading to lifestyle disorders, unstable blood sugars, constipation, sleepless nights, dull skin — the list is endless. Junk is junk, avoid it but don't badnaamofy carbs, at least not in our country where they are an integral part of our culture and cuisine.

Cooking traditions

And that brings me to another point: our traditional recipes and cooking. What's this whole fuss about boiled veggies and steamed veggies? What's so wrong with the tadka? The Indian style of cooking liberally uses hing, turmeric, jeera, sesame, curry leaves, green chillies and many other spices, condiments and herbs to give a dish its distinct flavour, aroma and taste. Now ask Tarla Dalal or Sanjeev Kapoor and they will tell you that food and the way you cook is an expression of divinity itself. It's an underrated art, and our own distinct style of cooking is a legacy worth preserving, documenting and practising.

Every region in our diverse country has its own distinct style of cooking. A north Indian's dal is different from a south Indian's, which differs from the Marathi dal and that of the Rajasthani and that of the Assamese. Now within this too, every community, caste, tribe, village will have its own 'secret' ingredient and recipe. It's just too bad that we have failed to package and market it as exotic, magical or 'fat-burning'. But don't let that take away from the fact that it actually is exotic, magical and fat-burning. Vir Sanghvi (I think he has brilliant insights on food, cooking, restaurants and the art of eating; plus, he looks good) wrote an article on how we are losing our local cuisine to global cuisine. Learning from the rest of the globe is always a good thing; adopting things which appeal to you is great; letting go of what you already have and what is useful (though not valued) is NOT.

This art of knowing exactly when to add the spices to the oil, or the science of how long you should heat the oil, or whether you put the hing first or the haldi is worth the effort because it aids digestion, assimilation, excretion, yes, but it also has anti-ageing, memory-sharpening, muscle-toning, fat-reducing and even cancer-preventing properties. But we will let go of this because we want to avoid calories or think yummy – fattening, yucky = lose weight, get thin quickly. Now you just boil the vegetable, or make it into a sabzi but not add the tadka, and eat it virtuously. Do you get all the fat-burning, anti-ageing, digestion-aiding, yummy-tasting and therapeutic properties of tazaa ghar ka khana? No, you get grief. So learn to enjoy life by learning to enjoy food. (Please don't confuse 'enjoy' with 'greed', dabaoing or sensory overload associated with stuffing your mouth.)

Filtered oil

So what about oils and frying — is that not 'fattening'? Not if you apply the three strategies mentioned above: use local oil, respect the rule of Uno (know where to stop), and involve yourself a bit in how your oil was made. We Indians use a lot of groundnut oil, ghee and in some regions sesame, til, safflower and sunflower oil. Now here's the thing, when you buy oil, look for the word 'filtered'. Filtered oil involves a process where the seed from which the oil is extracted is subjected to lower temperatures than 'refined' oils. So what does that mean for us? Lower temperature means less damage to the fat-soluble vitamins like A, D, E (rich in antioxidant properties), less damage to the molecular structure of fatty acid bonds in the seed (so more heart-protecting properties) and the need to use good quality seeds because of the smell and because impurities will not be destroyed at low temperatures (better seed = better aroma, flavour while cooking).

So do we use filtered oil made from our traditional methods, which use a wooden ghana or vessel and low temperatures? Not really. Two main contributing reasons for this: 1) They are not sold as 'heart-protecting and antioxidant rich', will retain some colour (often and wrongly associated with cheap or for 'poor people'), are not available in fancy bottles — basically poor packaging and marketing and 2) The high costs involved in making

oils the traditional way as the seeds w
their oil.

The economical way of making o...
solvents, high temperatures and technology to extract
every little bit of oil that can be squeezed from the seed.
And because the squeezing is so complete, you can use a
lower grade of seed. Now you have a really 'cheap' oil, or
better yield (more oil extracted per seed). The fancy bottles
that you find in supermarkets with 'added antioxidants
and vitamins' (they have to, their processes are killing the
naturally existing bonds and antioxidants, even changing
the molecular structure of bonds within the fatty acids by
a process called 'polymerisation' which can be potentially
damaging to the heart) are mostly the refined oils. They
also have tons of money to market and grab your 'mind
space' as heart-protecting oils. This is called 'yeda banke
pedha khaneka', Mumbaiya for pretentious attitude. So
people, **use 'filtered' or 'cold-pressed' or 'virgin' oils
to get the maximum nutrients from your oil.** Don't let
them go home with money earned from your ignorance.

Brown or white?

Shift to brown rice — heard that dictum before? Okay, chew
on this: white rice, where we pound the rice to remove its
outer covering, is not at all bad, in fact it's great. The bad
thing is when we mindlessly decide if one thing is good for us
and that if we do it a lot, it becomes only better. We do that
with rice so often now.

Every rice season, as we joined our ajoba (paternal
grandfather) in our farm in Sonave (outside Mumbai), we
would see women pounding, cleaning, shifting rice endlessly
from sunrise to sunset. Pounding rice removes the outer layer
of the rice, and with it part of the fibre and vitamin B too. Is
fibre and vitamin B good for you? Absolutely. So why are they

doing it? To remove the husk and bran, the outer part of the rice; but the protein, vitamin B and fibre *inside* the grain is still retained.

In fact, the protein in white rice is absorbed much better by your body than that in brown rice. It is also way easier to cook and digest white rice as compared to brown rice. Anywhere in India, when you are sick and down, what are your given? Khichdi. And khichdi has white rice, sweeties: it's easy to digest, easy to absorb, easy to assimilate proteins from and easier on your excretory system too. Ayurveda uses rice-based diets in treating various imbalances in the body. If rice that's devoid of its husk and bran is as 'fattening' as it's made out to be, all of our coastal belt would be floating in their backwaters (fat floats), but are they?

To get the best of both the worlds, polish your rice but not to the extent that it emits blinding whiteness. Remove the outer bran but allow the rice grain to show off its brown/red strains (this is what I refer to as brown rice, not the wrongly understood one with the husk and bran intact). No, don't worry, this won't compromise on the taste, and yes, you can totally eat your basmati with the red/brown strains too. This is exactly how the farming community of India eats their rice. Ever checked out their sizzling waists and six packs?

PS: Also, as India is dominantly vegetarian, getting proteins from rice, especially the essential amino acid methionine, branched chain amino acids and the conditionally essential (becomes essential under conditions of stress) amino acid tyrosine is crucial for us. So if you are vegetarian, stop fussing over rice all the more, just eat it.

PPS: You can eat rice even if you are diabetic. Chill. You need those proteins too.

Sweet visa

And what about sweets and desserts, won't they make us fat? No, not if you apply all strategies above, and then apply what I call as the rule of 'visa'. Stood in big queues for your US visa only to have it rejected by a rude officer? Then you know what I'm talking about. Big and strong nations don't hand out visas to all and sundry. They make their own evaluations (based on their own logic) and make decisions about who they consider 'worthy' of entry into their country. A weak nation, however, hands out visas quite liberally. So when it comes to your stomach, make it like a super-power nation, which decides not just the number of visas, let's say H1 visas, that will be handed out every year, but also who it will be handed out to. So the number of times you eat a dessert in the year should be strictly controlled like the H1 visa. If you've allotted thirty-six, twelve, fifty-two, whatever number (once a month, twice a month, and a day each of Diwali + one for birthday, anniversary, grandpa's eightieth whatever — up to you to decide), get prudent with it and hand it over to only 'worthy' occasions. So bad mood and feel like a pastry won't count as worthy, but 'first salary' or anything that's meaningful in your life gets the visa. Once you exhaust your allotted number you are not allowed to allot more visas. Also if you hand it over to 'unworthy' situations, it's your fault. See, the American embassy will take your paper almost two months prior to your interview. Take a leaf out of their book and take applications well in advance so that you can make thoughtful decisions on giving your 'sweet visa' to the right situation.

So as long as we eat according to the four principles and learn to apply the nutrition strategies, we don't need to kick ourselves over the occasional sweet or fried item. It's really not going to make us fat or destroy our diet; it is in fact accepted as part of our diet.

II

EXERCISE STRATEGIES

If you have an an ass, move it.
−Anonymous (or maybe I said it in one of my
bright moments)

What would you do if you were made prime minister for a day? 'I will build a huge sports complex,' she said, and there Madhu Sapre lost her chance to become Miss Universe in 1992. She was the front runner to win the crown, and she almost did, till she displayed her 'insensitivity' and actually said in so many words that she would build a sports complex. Here was a good-looking woman from a poor country like India: shouldn't she care about poverty, children and world peace? 'But then they asked us to speak straight from the heart (and not be politically correct), and in a year what can one do about poverty (anybody who comes from a poor country knows that), but a sports complex is doable and it can make the poor feel at par with the rich,' reasoned Madhu later. Sounds reasonable, right? But the bias against women and what they are supposed to feel sympathy for is universal, as universal as the concept of peace, love, harmony. Women constantly carry this burden of the assumption that we're supposed to put children, education, poverty, home, peace, etc. over our own health, fitness, wellness. The next time you feel that stabbing guilt when you make your way to the gym, reason with yourself: if I have to work at my best, mother at my best, play all the multiple roles I have chosen for myself with ease and without being tired and irritated, then I must invest my time wisely and spend time strengthening and nurturing my physical body.

Now I do know that most women will be left with very little time to themselves and then, of course, there are simply too many 'valid reasons' (read excuses) as to why we must postpone exercising to tomorrow/Monday/next month/next year and sometime after little Babloo starts going to school or maybe after he passes his 10th Std or whatever.

But I can't emphasise enough the need to stay physically fit and to indulge in regular, hardcore exercise. Women are exposed to many biologically challenging events: regular menstrual cycles, childbearing, rearing, nursing, and then sociological reasons like moving with the family and husband (often without having a say in the matter), learning to make compromises on every front (and without complaints), etc. We should be working out and keeping fit out of biological necessity and not out of some pressure to stay or look thin. However, it's often us women who, as little girls, will give up on exercising or simply running around the grounds, jumping, hanging on branches, twisting, shoving, pulling, pushing basically anything 'hardcore' (boyish/manly) the minute we reach puberty, which is such a shame, really! The minute girls in my building hit 7th-8th Std, they just start standing around in packs, and at the most do rounds of the building.

I think that's why Madhu Sapre wanted a sports complex. As an athlete, she understood the downside of the lack of facilities. Think about it, if you have parents paying for fancy club memberships, even then you have to rise above social conventions of what is considered 'boyish', or more 'important' (such as 10th/12th Std exams) and continue playing your sport. If your parents are not rich enough to buy memberships, what do you do, roam around the building or your mohalla? Wait to grow up to buy a membership is one option. You could rise above the social conventions of what is considered more important at your age (probably marriage/giving birth, etc.) and pursue a sport then. But the thing is, if you've been an active and fit teenager, then, a) you don't get fat during your shaadi/work/mothering periods and b) even if you do, your chances of getting back in shape and quickly are sky high.

We all have to realise that it is as important for our girls, daughters, mothers, sisters, aunts, grandmothers to indulge in hardcore physical activity and sports, as much as it is important for us to have womankind educated, literate and encouraged to pursue higher education. (You know how some families, specially the fathers-in-law, will khao bhav and tell everybody who is willing to listen that they insisted that the bahu finish her education and did everything to ensure that she can pursue it post marriage without any disturbance etc.? They need to talk about our fitness in the exact same vein. 'I told my bahu, no giving up on your game/gym/morning run/yoga.' Now I would give a million dollars to hear that [earn and give, of course ☺].)

Now I guess we all know how education affects and improves not just the life of the woman directly, but also that of her children, family, community or world at large. The exact same reasons are valid for women to remain physically fit. It's the physically fit who will be the leaders, game changers, thinkers, scientists, path-breakers. Yoga, running, weight-training, swimming, playing a game, dancing, group exercises — everything works (provided it fulfils the criteria listed further ahead in the section).

Equal opportunity

Invariably on our treks, after lunch, the boys will suggest playing a sport, usually cricket. They will draw great pleasure making bats out of a log of wood and making stumps out of some branches, hunt for a ball and have a blast playing. The girls (mostly women who are quite in shape) will only look on enviously. Most of these women are independent, as competent, or better than the men in their chosen fields, and invariably shouldering much more responsibility than the men in their lives. But when it comes to outdoor games, women have had to face the gross injustice of a lack of equal opportunity. Boys continue playing through their high school, into college etc., and at the most give up because of 'work hours'. Sadly, women give up playing sometime in high school, and then their 'work life' extends itself way beyond office hours. I know our parents (especially mothers) will be disturbed/lecture us if we don't study hard in school, worry about our dark future and difficult life. What is their response if we don't play hardcore during these years? How many mothers have been genuinely upset that their girls are no longer playing a sport? Are they even aware of the dangers looming in their girls' futures if they don't play? They are darker than not getting admission in a specific college for a specific course. These dangers will prevent the girls from enjoying life to its optimum and, worst case scenario, could lead to fatal conditions. Rise and shine mothers, it's up to you — push your girls hard, push them to exercise, push them towards physical learning and push by setting a fine example.

The funny part is women trek just as well as the men, so physical fitness is not really the issue, the issue is deeper — that of discrimination. Since a trek is a space for equal opportunity, both genders do well and the ability to enjoy it to the fullest is not hindered by discrimination.

Kinesthetic intelligence

When an old aunt slips in the bathroom, she falls and in all probability suffers a fracture and has to be helped out of the bathroom. When a young child slips in the bathroom, she gets joy out of the feeling of sliding on the slippery wet bathroom floor. She probably doesn't crash down to the floor, but even if she does, she almost never suffers a fracture, much less need any rescue effort. The act of falling is the same, the same bathroom, the same degree of wetness, slipperiness, etc., then why does the aunt suffer a fracture and the child only enjoy the feeling of falling? The answer is kinesthetic intelligence: the child has the body intelligence to know which muscles to contract, which ones to relax, which joint to flex, which one to extend, to prevent the fall; and if she does fall, she has the intelligence to know how to take it while minimising the load or weight on her joints. So even before she falls, she stands up. If you have seen Jonty Rhodes fielding at the point, then you know what I am talking about. On more than one occasion it seems like he is going to crash into the stumps or break one of his bones or at least strain, sprain or pull a muscle. No, sorry, his kinesthetic intelligence is just sky-high. My favourite sports picture is of Jonty Rhodes parallel to the floor at the height of the stumps, with his arm extended and the ball hitting the bails; the caption reads: It's a plane, it's a bird, it's JONTY RHODES!

Okay, okay, I know you have no plans of being a cricketer and much less Jonty Rhodes, but if you want to look sexy, toned, youthful and energetic, and not suffer fractures in your old age because of falls, or a backache because of a long flight, or cramps in the calf after a day of wearing stilettos, then you need to pay attention to kinesthetic intelligence. And for this, just like you go to school sincerely and dedicatedly without missing it for a day, you have to regularly play, work out, dance, practice martial arts — basically anything that employs the body, its nerves, joints, muscles, bones, organs, etc. Use your body and use it regularly to keep it in great shape. To give another example, remember how about five-six years ago, in the good old days, each one of us could remember at least ten phone numbers by heart? Now with mobile phones and their memories, we don't even remember our partner's, parent's or office phone number. Use it or lose it.

Five subjects of the workout paathshala

Let's assume that there is a workout school out there that you could attend. You'd be taught five main subjects: cardio-respiratory fitness, muscular endurance, muscular strength, flexibility and body composition. You cannot do any justice to the time spent working out or the calories burnt if they do not lead to any kind of progress or learning in these five core areas of fitness.

Cardio respiratory fitness: Ability of the heart and lungs (also called as cardio-pulmonary fitness) to deliver oxygen and nutrients to working cells or muscles which are demanding them. Let's say you're climbing stairs:

your leg muscles will demand more blood supply, oxygen and nutrient delivery, and will need to remove or recycle waste products (like lactic acid).

Muscular strength: The greatest amount of force (maximal effort) that a muscle or a group of muscles can exert at one time. Ever watched a cop lagao a lafa? That's muscular strength. Or when Sunny Deol says, 'Yeh dhai kilo ka haath jab padta hai to aadmi uthta nahi, uth jata hai'. The technical term in exercise physiology is 'one rep max' but apna Bollywood describes it better.

Muscular endurance: The ability of a muscle or a group of muscles to perform repeated activity over a period of time. For example, if you're moving furniture or if you're making laddoos, then you'll be using your muscular endurance.

Flexibility: Ability of the joints to move through their full range of motion (ROM). For example, a bowler would move her arm through a full range of motion of her shoulder before the delivery.

Body composition: This refers to the fat mass that you carry as compared to the total body mass you have. For women this should be twenty-five per cent or under. So even if you weigh a hundred kilos, not more than twenty-five kilos should come from fat. When women say they want to look toned and not flabby, they actually mean that they would like to reduce the fat mass and increase their lean mass (bone and muscle).

Now, the moral of the story is when you make improvements on the first four parameters of fitness, it results in an improvement (lowering fat mass) in the fifth parameter, that of body composition. Learning these 'subjects' or making improvements on these fitness parameters leads to an improvement in overall health, sense of well-being, sharpens your kinesthetic intelligence and, ya, improves your appearance as well. It also leads to perfect harmony in our hormones, stable moods and puts the mind into 'feel good' mode, unlike the high-strung or run-down state of mind that most weight loss plans lead to.

One of the reasons why I call the book 'weight loss tamasha' is exactly this. **No one seems to talk about getting fitter, sharpening the kinesthetic intelligence, improving quality of life, increasing the well-being quotient, etc.** All that we seem to care about is losing inches and getting that needle on the weighing scale to move down. Any weight loss or inch loss achieved without an improvement on the five fitness parameters above is a tamasha, a joke, cheating, a criminal waste of time, money and resources. What are we thinking when we buy into those 'two months, five kilos' (buy fifteen kilos and get three kilos free for any family member — my favourite ad), 'seven sessions, nine kilos' guarantees, one week 'detox' before shaadi, etc.? If we don't think about asking questions like, will it make my knees stronger, bones denser, skin smoother, hair thicker, mind calmer, hunger signals sharper, etc., then we deserve the diets we get, pretty much like we deserve the politicians we get because we don't ask them the right questions or give a damn for accountability (other than living room conversations of course).

So let's understand this well. Weight loss is a by-product (but not essential) of an improvement in body composition, which in turn is an essential by-product of improvement in the first four parameters of fitness. If you want to save your skin literally (sagging, wrinkles) and figuratively, then you must opt for fitness and weight loss programmes that are not sold or popular for 'weight loss'. Samjha? Don't buy into programmes that say 'pay x and lose y kilos'. Also, don't go under the knife to lose weight. Simply because weight lost at the cost of a decrease in all five core fitness parameters (which is what most 'diets', 'procedures', 'surgeries', 'toning tables', 'techniques', 'herbal or ayurvedic pill/ potions' do), is simply worthless.

And no, these five areas of fitness are not meant only for athletes or sports persons, they are meant for people like you and me, the ones who do a lot of sitting around and lead sedentary lifestyles. Athletes or sportspersons need these five core areas and then build on other parameters specific to their sport, like agility, power, speed, hand-eye coordination, etc. Why am I telling you all this? Because I want to make sure that you don't tell yourself that this is for sports people/size zero/youngsters/celebs etc. **This is for all of us and we can improve at any age, at any weight.** These are the very basic foundations of nurturing the physical body to use it like a vehicle fit to pursue higher goals of human life (the Vedic tradition, in fact all religious traditions adhere to this view). No higher purpose can be achieved when you lose those two or twenty kilos or fit into a size six or whatever, but it can be when you have enough energy and enthusiasm left at the end of your day. Incidentally, this is also how exercise science describes physical fitness: to go through day-to-day activities without feeling unduly tired and to have enough energy left to tackle emergencies, pursue hobbies, exercise or higher spiritual goals.

Learn to take time off

I had signed up for an intensive yoga course at my ashram in Netala. Just six days into the course, the asana, pranayama and bandha practice three times a day, and waking up at unusually early hours, left me feeling sick, tired and feverish. On the seventh day, I skipped the early morning prayer and chanting session and lay in bed, sleeping. By 6.30 a.m., my roomies returned to the dorm to pick up their mats and stuff for the asana practice that would start by 7 a.m. Startled, I woke up feeling guilty about missing the early morning class and miserable about not having enough self-discipline. I gave myself a pep talk on why I was there and how I had to optimise my time and learn everything that I could in these fifteen days and blah blah. Fully charged now, I got dressed, rolled up my mat, carried my notebook and braved my way to the asana hall by the Bhagirathi river. 'Where are you going Rujuta?' asked my teacher, Swami Govindananda, blocking my way at the entrance of the hall. 'To the class, Swamiji,' I replied, with a sense of pride and dignity. 'With fever?' he asked. 'Yes, I already missed the morning class and can't miss more, I am here to learn.' 'Good then learn this, go back to your dorm.'

I thought the swamiji would be proud of me for having the courage to fulfil my 'responsibility or obligation' to attend morning practice. I also thought he would be disappointed/ upset with me for sleeping in late during a course. Instead here he was, blocking my way to the entrance hall and not a wee bit angry. Dejected and miserable I walked back to the dorm. I just couldn't figure out why he was acting the way he was. He followed me and said, 'Come let's sit in the garden, and bring your shawl.' I obeyed. 'Swamiji, why?' I asked when I was in the garden, watching my course-mates getting into serious asana practice while I sat twiddling my thumbs and swinging my legs aimlessly. 'Because you have a fever, it's your body's way of saying "no asana practice today".' 'That's it?' I asked rudely, feeling let down by my body. 'So

I go through nine hours of practice for six days and on the seventh day I have fever? I am really so disappointed with my body.' 'Why? You should be grateful to her. Grateful that she is kind enough to tell you what her limits are. Good that you get fever, or else you will not learn to respect the body's limitation and even less learn how to overcome them.

'So take the day off, week off, whatever time the body needs to adapt and don't work against your body, work with her. She does whatever you want from her. Do you ever do a nine-hour practice in Mumbai?' 'No, not even ninety minutes.' 'Then, first thank the body that whenever you bring up a nine-hour practice, for six days she can keep up with the demand and only asks for a day's rest.

'Maybe this time your lesson here is this — learning to be grateful to your body for showing you her limits, being happy with yourself that you have the courage to push your body to the limits, and more importantly to stop at the first sign or demand to slow down. This is the only way both you and your body can learn.' My disappointment was replaced with gratefulness and once more I thought to myself how unlimited access to committed and experienced teachers is so important. No wonder the gurukul system produced finer students and individuals compared to our 7 a.m. to 2 p.m. or noon to 6 p.m. schools.

The day before, I had 'read' that when the body is tired, has fever for example, there should be no asana practice, according to the Hatha yoga pradipika. It could harm you and weaken your nervous system. But had I learnt to bring that into practice? No, not until the morning I woke up sick.

So why am I telling you all this? Because it really makes sense to not work out when you are tired mentally or physically and it makes no sense to push yourself when all you should do is skip and chill.

The principles of exercise

To make the most improvement in these five areas, we need to follow the guidelines or principles of exercise. These are rules that will make your exercise routine effective, i.e., will enable you to burn fat during and after exercise and ensure progress, learning and sharpening of your kinesthetic intelligence.

1. Progressive overload principle, often called the mother of all training or exercise principles. This means that the stress or stimuli that you put your body through during training should be greater than what you normally encounter in your day-to-day activities and should increase in an incremental order.

This is one reason why 'walking' doesn't qualify as exercise. You walk from your bed to the bathroom or from your car to the lift. So when you go for a 'walk', you are not exactly overloading the system and therefore the benefits that you achieve on your five core fitness parameters are limited. Now read the name of the principle again: PROGRESSIVE overload principle. This means that even if you choose to walk as a means of exercise, then you must progressively learn to do more during your walk. For example, run for some time in between the walk, or try walking the same distance in less time.

2. Specific Adaptation to Imposed Demands (SAID). A crucial principle to your fitness routine, this one is based on the most basic ability in us humans — the ability to adapt. Simply put, it means that our body and all its systems (nervous system, our circulatory system, cardio-pulmonary system, skeletal system, basically every system and metabolic pathway) adapt to the specific demands or stresses that we put on them. Ever wondered why you only find certain species of animals in certain latitudes on Earth, but humans can live anywhere from the North Pole to the South Pole? SAID is at work, humans adapt.

So a Ladakhi would have a system adapted and therefore 'suitable' to altitude, while a Keralite will have a system that can dissipate heat better and help her deal with humidity and heat. It also means that the Keralite will get mountain sickness in Ladakh and a Ladakhi will get sea sickness in Kerala, ha ha ha, kya PJ mara hai!

Coming back to what we are really talking about. Basically, what this means is that, when you 'warm up' on the treadmill before a resistance or weight-training session, you falter on the SAID principle and will expose your body to injuries. To help your body perform better at resistance or weight-training, your warm-up should consist of weight- or resistance-training but at a lower intensity than your main workout. So if your 'main set' is 10 lbs for 15 reps, then the warm-up can be 5 lbs for 5 reps. It also means that your warm-up should be specific to the muscles used during the workout. If you're training your back, the warm-up should be for the back and not for the chest, get it?

The progressive overload comes before SAID, because without overload, adaptation cannot take place. It also means that if the overload is too little or too much, then injury, boredom or a plateau effect occurs.

3. Recovery. This comes after SAID, because whether or not you will adapt depends entirely on whether or not you will recover. I hope you're getting this: first you must choose the right stimuli (exercise) to overload (not more, not less) then you must recover from this stimuli to allow adaptation to occur. When recovery is compromised, adaptation doesn't occur; it means you don't make progress on the five core areas and therefore you are wasting your time burning those precious calories. Good recovery means good nutrition + hydration + sleep. So if you really want that fab body, eat right, drink right, sleep right. No shortcuts. This is also why I often say that eating right and working out are like two sides of the same coin. Only exercise, and being careless about eating right = lack of recovery = zero or at best limited result = frustration. Eating right but not working out = no overload = zero or limited result = frustration.

4. **Regularity**. Ha, ha, this is my personal favourite. The use it or lose it funda is based on this. The SAID principle leads to us having something called as 'muscle memory', much like brain memory. So if you are not regular with your workouts, you will go through something called as 'detraining' or 'de-conditioning'. Essentially, it means that your body will lose its kinesthetic intelligence and will get poorer at the five core areas of fitness. Gosh! Sounds like a nightmare. So if you wanna look sharp, toned, sexy, then train (exercise) with regularity. Read *regularity*, and not *daily*. Just ensure that you use all the previous three principles first to get the max out of your workout. Let me explain. You walk daily but don't care for overload = no improvement in the fitness parameters = kya time ka khoti! You train hard, almost kill yourself in the gym and then eat late night and don't sleep on time, so no recovery – no improvement on the fitness parameters – aunty, sudhar jao!

God, digressing again. I was making the point of muscle memory. This refers to nerves per unit of muscle fibre or the neural pathway your muscles will use to bring about an action. See, your right hand (or left, if you're a leftie) gets used frequently so you are stronger, sharper or can write with ease with that hand. The other hand doesn't get used regularly, so it is weak and can't write. Let's say you are thirty and attempting to write a three-hour paper when the last time you took an exam like that was when you were fifteen. Now, when you begin writing, the right hand will hurt at first but will slowly refresh its memory of writing exams and will eventually write like a pro. But the left hand still won't be able to write because it lacks the 'memory'.

Or let's say you were training regularly, then shaadi, baccha-kachha and it's been ten years since you exercised, but within weeks of starting to exercise again your body will ignite its muscle memory and bring your fitness parameters to where you last left them.

All in all, people with accumulated fitness or those who have a history of keeping fit will find it easier to make gains on the core fitness parameters when they start using the principles above. So women, don't let your past get in the way of your present and say, 'I used to be so fit and now look at me'. Simply start and in no time you will be back to your original fitness levels.

Word of caution: detraining can occur in about three weeks, so don't go without exercise for over three weeks, okay? It's very expensive metabolically for your body to maintain 'conditioning' or high levels of core fitness parameters, so if your body doesn't get the right stimuli to maintain it, it will bring the cost down and lower its metabolic spending. Bole ga toh, 'conditioning' means your first four core fitness parameters are well developed so your body will be leaner and fitter, carrying more muscle as compared to the fat it carries. Muscle is metabolically active tissue, it forces the body to burn fat to maintain itself, so if the muscles are not being used, the body will reduce spending on its fat tissue and detrain or lose the muscle tissue. Getting it? Low BMR = more body fat.

5. Principle of balance or variation. This simply means that the first four fitness parameters must be stimulated, adapted, recovered and trained regularly. In other words, if you only build strength and ignore flexibility or only work on cardio and ignore strength, then instead of getting fitter you will lose out on fitness and increase the chances of getting injured. Basically there are no short cuts. The next time somebody says 'just start walking' as a solution to your fitness, tell them that it won't address all the fitness parameters and therefore is not the 'best' exercise. Also, remember the next time somebody says 'use variation or you will not get results', it is coming out of a misunderstanding of the principle of variation or balance. You need to use a variety of exercises because you need to develop and stimulate various parameters of fitness. It doesn't mean a mindless switching from yoga to aerobics to weight-training. You need to build a well-rounded or complete (that which includes all the parameters) fitness programme, planned and executed based on the core training principles.

Adiponectin

Dr Len Kravtiz, an exercise physiologist, described it as a 'good guy hormone' at a fitness conference I attended in NYC. This hormone is secreted by the fat cells in the body. The leaner (lower fat weight and higher bone and muscle weight) and fitter you are, the more the adiponectin your fat cells produce. Adiponectin prevents occurrence of the metabolic syndrome that is associated with a higher risk of osteoporosis, high blood pressure, heart disease, diabetes, etc. See we need body fat; fat protects us from all the 'obesity'-related diseases by secreting the 'good guy hormone'. All we need is to support our fat cells with adequate bone and muscle tissue. Good news? Promise to stop pinching your thighs with contempt and work on improving your lifestyle instead. Want some more good news? Adiponectin also helps you reduce cellular inflammation, what we commonly refer to as 'bloating'. So just get fitter darlings.

III

SLEEP STRATEGIES

'Not everything that can be counted counts, and not everything that counts can be counted.'

–Albert Einstein

Einstein could well have been talking about the association of body weight and sleep. Body weight and weight loss can be counted but doesn't count for much (when it comes to your health, fitness and peace), as you have by now (fingers crossed) understood, but sleep does. Sadly, sleep can't really be quantified or qualified, or at least it's complicated to do so. But you can experience and know for sure that when you don't sleep well, your recovery suffers, you wake up tired, feel bloated, lethargic and generally are like a zombie, and bust goes your exercise and diet plans or at least they get pushed to the next day. This is clearly the most overlooked and underappreciated aspect of 'weight loss' (fat loss, improved body composition). (Like how a housewife's contribution to running an efficient kitchen and home pushes the husband's business profits higher; you can't prove it, but you *know* there is a strong link and you wish there were a conclusive way to prove it.)

Lack of sleep, and I mean good quality sleep, will push your diet and exercise plans to the next day, therefore keeping you FAT for today, and could even lead to a host of lifestyle and metabolic disorders like PCOS, thyroid malfunction, diabetes, high blood pressure, osteoporosis etc., basically keeping you from expressing your potential and enjoying your life to the fullest.

Overeating followed by long gaps between meals (an underlying factor in gaining body fat) is not a vicious cycle, it's a downward spiral, and lack of sleep contributes to it. When you wake up tired and groggy you need a stimulant to wake you up so you have a cup of coffee/tea, and from there on begins the atyachar on your digestive system. You lose touch with the hunger signals your body's sending you, will eat nothing for up to four hours (or more) and eventually end up gobbling every morsel that flies past you. If you decide to give in to the feeling of 'five minutes more', you end up sleeping much longer (always) and then have difficulty sleeping in the night. Staying up at night is the prequel to midnight snacking. So deviyon, waking up fresh is the only option and forms a non-negotiable Strategy 3 to lose weight.

I really can't over-emphasise the importance of a restful night; to be able to sleep at will is nothing short of a blessing. 'Gudakesh' is one of the names by which Sri Krishna calls Arjuna in the *Bhagvad Gita*. It means somebody who is so powerful that he has gained control over sleep. Arjuna could sleep (and stay awake) at will. One must not eat or sleep too much (or too little) is one of the messages of the *Gita*, and religions world over have the same message — that it is important to be disciplined about sleeping and eating if one is to enjoy and actualise the vast human potential. For now we will limit this to the human potential to lose weight.

In our 'modern' (messed up) life, human intelligence is used to create flat screen TVs which can be watched lying down, and thick curtains can be employed to block sunlight from entering your bedroom and disturbing you from the deep sleep that you invariably fall into in the early hours (between 6-9 a.m.) of the morning. The SAID principle (see Exercise Strategy) works boss, wherever you employ it, so your body adapts to the TV, thick curtains in the bedroom and quickly gets rid of 'unwanted' (lean) tissue of the body and gets fat as a response to the sedentary lifestyle.

To reverse the damage (or adaptation), we need to undo what we have become used to and take the following steps:

1. No TV in the bedroom. Ya, I know you can afford a flat screen and it has BEE rating and that it is blah blah blah, but come on, it's not worth it ladies. Not when that fat pops over the sides of your jeans and right on top of your zipper. I told you earlier na, the bigger the TV, the bigger the size of your jeans, the flatter the TV, the rounder your stomach. God, I think I am a walking, talking Ramsay film, sounds like a horror story na?

Hindustani classical music is one of the things that we all will bhav maro on (specially in front of firangs or when in phoren), but will give a damn about when it comes to actually applying or practising this wisdom (yes sweety, it's wisdom not just art) in our daily lives. Music originates from the Sama ved, and in classical music certain ragas are meant to be listened to at particular times. Heard about ratri ka pehla prahar, dopahar ka doosra prahar etc., right?

So much for the Vedic culture, sanskriti, sabhyata if we 'unwind or sleep' listening to random, loud, screeching noises from the TV. The news anchors are not talking in the sur or sargam that's recommended for 'ratri ka prahar' nor are the saas, bahus, bechari betis or akha parivaar or whatever you watch. On the one hand we would like to take digs at the Ekta Kapoor (I feel we should add 'the' before her name, she is the TV empress, easily) or find *Peepli Live* a great satire, but on the other hand we will lap up anything they dole out to us and we will do it daily. So who is the joke on? Ekta Kapoor, media, or on you ma'am?

Watching and hearing sounds from TV robs you of restful sleep that is oh so essential for fat loss. 'Oh! I wonder how she goes to sleep every night.' If you have ever said that about somebody who's going through a rough period in her life, or has done some lafda like chori or extramarital affair, or forgotten to pick up her daughter from school one day, etc. (ya, ya, we are such judgmental bitches), then remember that lights and sounds in the night emitting from the TV, laptop, playstation are stressful and qualify as an offence too. Yes, you are cheating your biological clock, and if I were you and nursed dreams of fitting into a tight choli and wearing a saree three inches below my navel, arrey baapre, I wouldn't ever dare to cheat my biological clock. Here's why.

The biological clock

The biological clock (the suprachiasmatic nucleus or SCN)

is a tiny little mungi-sized structure which has haathi-sized effects on weight loss. It is located in the hypothalamus region, contains over 20,000 neurons and is strategically placed at a point where it can stay in constant touch with the optic nerves. So your eyes constantly tell the SCN whether it's day or night or twilight, etc. The SCN tells all other parts of your brain including the pineal gland what to do depending on the time. So if it's evening or night, the mungi will tell the pineal gland to secrete the hormone melatonin which will induce sleep. Now if your eyes have picked up the radiation from the TV (or the laptop) then — dhan te nan — no melatonin, let's activate catecholamines instead. Catecholamines are hormones which put your body in the fight or flight mode (opposite of inducing sleep; it induces feelings of alertness — ready to kill or die) and are secreted by the adrenal glands above your kidney. This group of hormones also interferes with another hormone called leptin, which is secreted by your fat cells and decreases its levels. Leptos is Greek for 'thin', so the levels of this hormone which induces satiety (prevents overeating and keeps you thin) and asks you to stop eating, goes down and your brain asks you to eat. Think about it: late-night movie and a bucket of popcorn — is the puzzle getting solved for you? So the ghar ka equivalent of watching TV before sleeping or having it in the bedroom with the 'adjusting' husband putting on ear phones to save you from the noise and the 'stubborn' wife getting exposed only to radiation = a wife who feels 'not full or wants something meetha' after a meal or 'feels like a pastry' in the night or 'sleep walks' to the fridge in the night. God! Even writing about it makes me sick!

So you want me to say it again? **Say NO to TV in the bedroom, say YES to the saree and wear it three inches below the navel.** Ha, ha, can I get a job as a copy writer? Guess not, so I will proceed to writing the second sleep strategy.

Sleep and intuition

'Where did you learn all this?' asked my little cousin Easha. The question was loaded with scepticism and directed towards Lamaji, our guide in Darma Valley, after someone declared he could fly if required. 'When I was small, I learnt in my dreams,' he answered in all earnestness. Easha looked at me with eyes that said: Main Alibag se aaya kya? The Mumbaiya equivalent of, 'I may still be in school but I am no fool'. I felt guilty because I believed Lamaji's story. The Bihar School of Yoga has worked extensively on exploring this 'I learnt in my sleep' thingy, they call it 'Yog Nidra' and have used its 'magical' powers to teach math tables to sleeping children or teach yoga to jail inmates. Can you learn or awaken your intuition in your sleep? Yes, it's been proved beyond doubt that sleep improves well-being, learning abilities and memory powers. August Kekule discovered the cyclic structure of Benzene in his sleep. Till he slept over it, nobody had ever thought that six carbon atoms could link to each other in any other way but in one straight line. By dreaming about six carbons in a hexagon or the cyclic nature of Benzene, as it is now popularly called, Kekule changed chemistry forever. Today when you read articles about how sleeping affects your hormones and therefore interferes with weight loss, spare a moment to thank him. Had it not been for his intuition about Benzene's true nature, you would have never figured out how lack of sleep leads to hormonal disturbances (your hormones have a lot of these cyclic structures) and how that affects your weight loss.

You may not believe that sleeping well awakens intuition, but you can continue reaping the benefits of better understood bio-chemistry. Did you just say, 'In your dreams'? Well, all I can say is, 'Sleep over it.'☺

2. No booze before sleeping. Hello! I know you only sip the choicest wines and can go without drinking for years but only 'drink socially' to keep others company, or to keep people's mouths shut, or to not appear like a party pooper, or to just enjoy a romantic dinner or whatever. (The funniest one I have heard is: 'Look I have to be a little tipsy to have sex with my husband. I can't stand him otherwise.) Yes, I know you are not exactly lying in a gutter every night because you are too drunk to go home. I know all that. I also know that you do vodka or the harder stuff only once in a while, and I know that you don't drink every day of the week. Yes, I know I am not talking to an alcoholic! But listen, I still think I should tell you about the alcohol and weight loss connection.

I have only been working for eleven years, and even in that span of time I have seen a dramatic rise in metabolic disorders in younger women, some younger than fifteen. The other thing that I have seen, is a dramatic rise in my clients' 'social drinking' and my gut tells me that there is a connection.

Alcohol is thought of as something that helps you fall asleep. Well, it's not entirely untrue. It does help you fall asleep, but prevents you from entering the REM or deep restorative stages of sleep. It's in these stages that our body carries out all the repair and restoration work of the body and mind. Okay, have you heard of the hypoxia or low oxygen levels and disrupted sleep? If you have ever been to Ladakh or know somebody who has been to Ladakh, then you have heard of altitude sickness or how they couldn't sleep for the first couple of nights? That's because the oxygen supply to the brain was not adequate so their sleep was interrupted and they kept waking up many times in the night. Alcohol does the exact same thing and is one of the reasons why you may not usually snore but will definitely snore on nights when you have had a drink or two. Snoring is a sign of poor or disturbed sleep. Now close your eyes and imagine somebody snoring next to you: is that somebody fat? We always associate snoring with fat people — why? Because disturbed sleep does lower your metabolism, making you stay fat.

Amongst many other things, alcohol reduces the levels of serotonin which helps you to feel calm and keeps your 'sugar cravings' under control. That glass of wine/vodka/rum/whatever it is, is again going to put you in the fight and flight mode and, equally bad, reduce your body's natural production of the growth hormone. It's going to create an environment in your body where you can't recover even though you slept like a log — come put your hands together and welcome the hangover. It's simply your hormones saying — I feel fatigued and dead tired.

Some more bad news? Well, if you have been working out regularly, then the alcohol destroys your endurance or stamina levels (you probably know that) and it reduces the levels of the hormone testosterone too. Say tata to toned muscles and strong bones and make friends with an expanding waist line. You really are a cool girl!

I sound like a bitch? Yeah, I feel like one too. Talking about alcohol makes me feel fatigued because that's the long-lasting feeling from booze, not the 'high', and tired women are always bitchy, right?

Shabana Azmi

The only time I have felt ashamed for talking about how alcohol is more harmful for women than men is when I was invited as one of the speakers to a conference on women's health organised by IAOH (Indian Association of Occupational Health). So this conference was arranged for doctors who work with women in corporations and I guess it forms a part of employee welfare, etc. Anyways, this was way back in 2005 and they had called Shabana Azmi, Leena Nair, Sukanya from IBM and me. I was clearly the least qualified to talk about women, the challenges they face in the corporate work culture and the toll it takes on their mental and physical well-being or the steps that need to be taken to curtail them, but of course I thought otherwise. Leena Nair, the only woman director of HLL, looked in great shape and spoke about the discriminatory policies that companies needed to change, especially the one related to parents' insurance. Until recently a woman could have her parents insured by the employer only as long as she was unmarried; a working man can have his parents insured irrespective of his marital status. Sukanya, who headed HR in IBM, spoke about how the biggest challenge they faced was that women often discriminated against themselves, had low self worth and thought themselves unworthy of positions. Shabana Azmi chose not to speak about working women's health at all. She stood at the podium and fultu scolded every doctor in that gathering for promoting and supporting female infanticide. 'When you don't let them live, should we trust you to keep them well once they are alive?' Whoa... Doctors are not used to such blatant tongue-lashings; conferences are, after all, ego-massage exercises. She then went on to read the statistics on female infanticide and how south Mumbai, the richer part of Mumbai, had the most shameful records.

Later as I sat by the window seat and made my way back home in the train, my memory oscillated between a Shabana Azmi I had met only a few months ago where she had almost choked laughing because she had run out of time while playing a game of dumb charades and failed to enact *Reshma ki Garam Jawani* or some such movie to her teammates and to the angry woman making us all squirm with hard facts about murdering foetuses. She held the doctors, mothers, families, working women (that included me) and society at large responsible for failing to stop this menace. So I decided that I was the best speaker because I stuck to the point and delivered a crisp talk on why alcohol (social drinking), cigarettes, tea and coffee are hazardous for working women and can have deadlier short and long term effects on them as compared to working men. Sukanya and Leena (I don't remember who I ranked second and third) came after me and the worst was Shabana Azmi. She had after all said everything I didn't want to hear.

God knows that if I am put back on the train today, I would think all these women, especially Shabana, made some strong valid points, with me making the least important ones. Yes, first we must let women live, then as a society we must eliminate discrimination against them, and then we must encourage them to stop discriminating against themselves. After all this, whether they stay thin or fat is really no big deal. The health hazards that working women face (we all work, it's just that some of us are compensated financially for a part of our work) are beyond that glass of wine or body weight. Sigh!

3. No dessert/pastry/sugar/tea/coffee — basically no stimulant — post sunset. Hmm... Now what can I tell you that you don't already know?

You know one of the things I absolutely hate is emails in my inbox from girly mags or Sunday newspapers asking me for examples of comfort food. Sample this:

Hi Rujuta,
Please send me very quickly answers to the following:
What are the comfort foods when feeling –
- *Bored*
- *Tired*
- *Lazy*
- *Cranky*
- *Fatigued*

*Will appreciate your quick response. I need answers in
detail by 3.30 p.m.*

I had received this email at 1.30 p.m., and no, it was
not from my boss or my mother-in-law; in fact it was
nobody I had ever met/interacted with before. The
only reason why this journo was throwing her weight
around (according to me ninety per cent of journos
are overweight) is because she worked for a 'most-read'
paper. But even less popular papers/mags (and less-paid
journos) will do this. **People who write about health
have nothing to do with it. I think this also contributes
to the rampant misinformation about food, exercise
and weight loss.** What's more, they have little or no
patience to understand anything about it.

Okay, I am done with whining and cribbing, so let's get
to the point.

For starters, there is NO such thing as COMFORT
FOOD. There definitely are depressed states of mind and
fatigued bodies which look for a 'quick fix', but there's no
way to quickly fix a tired mind and body and there are no
quick answers to that email either. You know, when you
see a woman dig into pastries or mithai or declare that
she has a sweet tooth, then, well, then you can assume
she is not getting enough action in bed! Oops, did I
just say that? Yes, I did and I stand by it. The tongue is
both a pleasure-giving and protecting organ. It tells you
what's good for you and what's not, doesn't it? If you are
eating something stale, it could be something beautifully
presented in a five star hotel, the tongue won't be fooled
by the eyes or the décor. It will declare, God! Is this dal
last night's leftovers? And come on, I can guarantee that

while you were digging into that sinful chocolate which overpowered your sense organs and the reasoning ability of your brain, your tongue declared — I shouldn't be eating this, or at least I should stop at two teaspoonfuls. See, the tongue protects, it tells you that overworking its pleasure centres is a crime. We have many pleasure centres, after all, right? Heard of genitals? Sorry, this book is for 'family reading' so let's put it this way: when the sexual organs are not nurtured it over-activates other pleasure centres. And eating too much sweet makes you dull, lethargic, unhealthy and fat and further reduces your chances of having sex.

The pleasure chakra

The swadhisthana chakra (remember it from the PCOD chapter? It's the chakra that not only controls or presides over your sexual desires, but also the desire to have more money or power) stays healthy and vibrant when one pursues money, power, sex meaningfully. So when I say 'not getting any action', I don't mean frequency, I mean purpose and meaning. Same goes with power and money — is it adding meaning to your life? If yes, you're in a good place.

What's more, the swadhisthana is involved with our creativity. The more labels we earn ('married', 'mother', 'working'), the less we pursue our hobbies — so no more Bharatnatyam, the sitar is fighting cobwebs, the badminton racket has been gifted to the bai, you no longer sing, not even in the bathroom, and you can't remember the last time you cooked for the sheer joy of it. So creativity is all stifled, drowning in worldly 'pleasures', leaving you no other option but to eat another chocolate post lunch! Tch tch. Grow up girls, let's make eating a pastry, mithai, chocolate a truly pleasurable activity where it doesn't send you on a guilt trip, not a minute after you eat, or hours later or the next morning.

The best way to ensure that eating mithai remains a sensory pleasure (and nothing else) is to not let it interfere with your sleep. Here's a simple formula you should by-heart (ha ha) — Sleep well = no sugar cravings in the day. Eat sweets after dark = lack of good quality sleep = sugar cravings the next day = lack of good sleep. (The same applies for tea, coffee or any other stimulant; I've only used 'sweets' because we tend to succumb to that craving much more often.)

After sunset, the body uses a neurotransmitter called GABA to reduce adrenaline and increase serotonin and dopamine, basically reduces your feelings of agitation and alertness and increases feelings of calm and peace. Eating a sweet or drinking a cup of tea/coffee has the exact opposite effect, i.e. you are buzzing at night. This makes you fat yes, but also does not allow you to sleep well, which then reduces your recovery and destroys your immune function and also reduces the levels of GABA itself. The lower the levels of GABA, the more the feelings of anxiety or depression (one of the reasons why people suffer from nightmares the night after a late dinner and dessert), and when we are anxious or low or depressed what do we reach out for? Sorry, you don't win any medal for the answer. I'm hoping, though, that you now understand that it's best to eat your 'treat' by 4 p.m. or before it gets dark.

4. No compensation. Okay, I am not going to bore you with details but I just want to put one point across: SLEEP CANNOT BE COMPENSATED FOR. So if you tell yourself you 'compensate' for a week's lack of sleep by oversleeping on weekends, or you need a vacation to 'compensate' for all the late nights you've had, or that you need to go to mom's to sleep and 'compensate' for all the Diwali partying, you are seriously fooling yourself.

Sleep should be automatic, just like waking up should be automatic. (Automatic like breathing. You are breathing right now, right? I mean effortless = automatic.) When sleep and waking up is automatic or effortless, going to the loo, eating on time, eating right, looking fab, glowing skin, lustrous hair, pink nails, strong immune function, protection from lifestyle diseases etc. is automatic or an absolutely given. Following the first three sleep strategies will empower you to never ever needing to 'compensate' for sleep.

In fact, all the sleep strategies can be written as just one strategy: 'NO snooze' or ' NO alarm'. If you need an alarm to wake up, or worse need to put the alarm on the snooze mode, know that you are not respecting your body's need to sleep. Waking up fresh is not a dream, it's a reality and it's so worth working towards that reality.

Sleep and appetite

Leptin and ghrelin are hormones associated with your appetite. Leptin, secreted by fat cells, makes you feel full and asks you to stop eating further, while ghrelin, secreted by your GI tract, makes you feel hungry and urges you to eat. You need both to work well in order to stay fit, and these two need you to sleep well to function at their best. Not following the basics of the Sleep Strategy will lead to over-secretion of the hormone ghrelin in the night. You may think you're eating late or raiding the fridge just to kill time, but it's actually a result of excess ghrelin or the hunger hormone. Then you keep going to the loo, and again you think this is only because you are unable to sleep, but the reality is the leptin levels have gone down. Leptin works along with other calming hormones to ensure that you sleep undisturbed. But with low levels of calming hormones in the night, you experience what is often called as 'disturbed sleep' (sleeping but still not asleep), and it's this disturbance that stresses every part of your body and raises your body temperature so you go to the loo to pee in the hope of lowering the body temperature. What a waste of energies, na?

What's worse is, when you do this routinely, over months or years, the body gets resistant to leptin, which means you are producing adequate leptin but it can no longer do its work of giving you the satiety signal, asking you to stop eating or calming you down. So you get into a pattern of never feeling content or satisfied with whatever or no matter how much you eat. This leads to chronic overeating or eating something sweet post a meal. End result — more body fat than you can handle.

Chalo, have you understood how lack of sleep leads to an increase in episodes of overeating? Leptin resistance. To keep the appetite healthy (the ability to know when to eat, how much to eat and when to stop eating), you've got to ensure that ghrelin and leptin work, and to do that, all you've got do is sleep on time.

Bedroom etiquette

- Keep the bed a place exclusively to sleep, nothing else. Don't eat there. Keep the laptop, Blackberry, books away from it.
- Move your TV to another part of the house, and if that's not possible, switch it off while having dinner and one hour prior to bedtime.
- You need the body temperature to go down a bit to ensure a restful sleep, so keep the windows open and the bedroom well ventilated. If you need to use an AC, then set the temperature right so that you are not waking up to switch the AC off or fan on multiple times in the night.

- If you have trouble sleeping, avoid exercising after sunset because your body temperature goes up and metabolism picks up after exercise, which can keep you from falling asleep.
- Use curtains that allow sunlight to reach your bedroom so that your bio clock wakes you up naturally and activates your brain to pick up your metabolism and alertness levels too.
- Use natural and non-synthetic pillow covers, bed sheets, etc. Your skin should be able to breathe while sleeping. Synthetic covers or that satin lingerie/night dress can upset your body's temperature regulation and interfere with sleep. Also change the bed sheets every two days. (Our body drops dead cells during the night.)
- Burn a nice, relaxing aroma oil to soothe your senses. Open the windows of your bedroom often. Air and sun bathe your bedding, don't just let it lie in the 'storage under the bed'.
- Bring back mosquito nets in place of chemical repellents.
- Above all, always go to bed at a fixed time. Okay, at least on most days of the week, sleep at a fixed hour.

IV

RELATIONSHIP STRATEGIES

If an Italian woman finds out her husband is having an affair, she will kill the other woman; a Spanish woman will kill her husband, and the Indian woman will kill herself!

–An old joke

See, an Indian woman will kill herself for just about anything, including losing weight. Uff! Teri adaa… Milk spilled? Bai extending leave without notice (yet again)? Father-in-law found too much masala in the food? Mother-in-law sulking because you left your cup on the table after drinking coffee? Mannu/Minni missed school bus by a whisker? Husband left dirty underwear for public display in the bathroom? Weight not budged in the last two weeks? God! I feel like killing myself! So the first thing we need to work on is our relationship with ourselves.

The need of the hour is for us to cultivate patience and forgiveness towards ourselves, to free ourselves from the unrealistic expectations we impose on ourselves, to learn to be our 'real' selves (not ideal). A REAL woman will put a hundred per cent effort towards all her responsibilities and KNOW that a hundred per cent effort is not equal to a hundred per cent result and an IDEAL woman doesn't exist. So stop chasing the unreal and get real. The real self is always happy, the unreal self is always searching for happiness and feeling lost. Also, getting fat and then unrealistically believing that losing weight will make you happy (or healthy) ... ha ha ha — what a cruel joke!

Obsessing with food and one's body, its shape, size and weight is a foolproof way of staying fat and unfit forever. Obsession with eating is now widely recognised as 'oral craving', a manifestation of some much deeper unresolved emotion. Ever noticed how eating too much at one time (often followed by long periods of starvation or 'detox') upsets your breathing? Invariably the breathing becomes faster, shorter, shallower, much like how it gets when you feel angry or upset. The breath is the link to the mind, when the breath is disturbed, so is the mind. When the breath is slow, soft, long, deep, the mind feels calm and at ease.

The Upanishads say that the diseases (getting fat is a disease dahlings, but NOT a crime) you create for yourself can be cured by yourself. And the Dalai Lama said, 'Problems cannot be resolved at the same levels of awareness that created them'. Samjha kya? You need to go from the level of being an ideal woman to a real woman if you must get healthier, happier (ya, ya to lose weight too).

So here are some strategies that will help you:

1. With great power comes great responsibility — Spiderman said that. Now if the guy who goes around with a mask over his face can understand that, what's wrong with us? I mean, look at us women and the number of responsibilities we have. Do we have the power or access to resources which will help us fulfil our hajjar responsibilities — the access to education, healthcare, sanitation, family planning? If yes, then we must use this power to become more responsible towards ourselves. In a country like ours, you are a rare species if you said 'yes' to the above. Most of the Bharatiya naris will say 'no' or will have limited access depending on the whims of the current most powerful person in their lives (father/husband/mother-in-law).

As a country, we have our problems, the cruellest being chronic hunger. Millions of Indians go hungry daily and a large number of them will die because of malnourishment. The biggest irony is that women like you and me, who have access (unlimited or limited) to resources will go hungry too, in the hope of losing weight. And if not totally hungry, we will invent so many fads and fears about food that we drive ourselves nuts: can't have peanuts; can't have rice at night; can't have puris; can't have … can't have … god! Food nourishes, let's you live, helps you carry out your responsibilities. And we've got that bonus, that we can study as long as we want, choose to reproduce when we want and have a bathroom which is not just clean, away from prying eyes but also practically designer. So now what? You have everything which ensures that you will NEVER be malnourished and yet you do everything that makes you malnourished. Yes, those vitamin B12, vitamin D3, iron, calcium deficiencies are screaming MALNOURISHMENT. Taking shots and popping pills doesn't work; being more responsible, getting more real and simple with food does.

How does this make its way to relationship strategies? How much and how well we eat is a sign of how much we value ourselves. All that power over reproduction, education, sanitation without self-worth is called … I don't know what it's called but, okay, undeserving, for the lack of a better word. Women are secondary citizens in our country but women like you and me have the power to at least at the personal level end the discrimination. Eat, and eat bindaas and at the time you need food, not after children are sent to school, dabba is made for husband, father-in-law finishes eating etc. Get it?

2. Debugging sucks, testing rocks (seen in the Google India, Hyderabad office loo). In the IT industry, if there's a problem with the program you've written, then you need to rewrite or recreate that program — a huge hassle and a time-consuming task. The process is called debugging. A much more effective thing to do is 'testing': check for everything that can go wrong and make a provision to ensure that it doesn't. Testing may appear time-consuming, but in fact it saves not just time, but also a lot of hassle. What's more, it makes you look smart. You've already checked and rechecked for all failures and plugged all the loopholes — what a smart girl you make!

Now use this great strategy and apply it to all your relationships, including that with food. So you decided to eat right, what can go wrong? You may not find dahi at 4 p.m.; you may run out of poha or oil to make breakfast; you forgot to take that calcium tablet at night; your colleagues may eat all your peanuts; you will only be offered biscuits or at best a sandwich at that working lunch meeting. So then what? If you start debugging or fixing the problem after it has already occurred, it sucks. Since you are one hell of a rockstar, or at least want to look like one, you must anticipate everything that can go wrong before it does and have back-up options; it's called testing and it's rocking.

Initially you may need to do testing on a daily basis, later weekly and over a period of time it will become an integral part of you. You won't even notice that you are testing, just like you don't even notice that you ate lunch late again today. Some tips for testing:

- Before going to sleep, decide what you will be eating for breakfast and check if the kitchen has everything you need to make it. Make a checklist: gas – check, poha – check, oil – check, herbs, spices, masala dabba – check, coconut – check, etc.
- Fix the days when you will go to your local bhaji market and buy veggies for not more than three days. Don't use the fridge as a store room and use a cloth bag to ferry your stuff. Walk to the market: that way you can burn calories and save parking time and petrol costs.
- If all you get is biscuits for meetings, bark (dogs eat biscuits) at the HR/management. Employee welfare means access to nutritious food, not coffee machines, biscuits and chips in the pantry and a smoking booth.
- Ensure that your handbag has two food options in it at all times.
- Keep your vitamins and minerals in a place where you can see them, that way you won't forget to take them. Investing in a fancy pill box works well too: that way you can have it in your handbag at all times.
- Decide at the breakfast table what your 4-6 p.m. meal is going to be and arrange it before stepping out of the house. Ya baby, you are not alone; we all eat wrong during that golden two-hour period. Actually we should be eating dinner around that time.

3. Pain is our friend. It tells us that something is wrong and needs to be corrected. When the children's homework, husband's TV viewing, mother-in-law, friend's bickering, standing for a long time becomes a pain, it's actually shouting CHANGE. In our current relationship with ourselves, we have learnt to put up with or brave the pain. Eating too late in the night, drinking more than two cups of tea/coffee in the day, grabbing breakfast, skipping lunch, and dabaoing dinner is painful (whether you do it once or all the time) — but do we change? No, we are such lazy girls that we'd rather blame our relationships with other people than change our own eating habits. 'What to do, my husband comes back home so late.' You must have heard that before, right? Why do you eat so late? My husband comes back so late! God! But you are at home, didn't you see yourself? Are you invisible? Become visible in your own eyes, allow your most basic need to eat become visible, so visible that it's difficult to not see that you are hungry while carrying out your 'responsibilities' or while trying to get 'thin.'

4. Okay, stomach this: **the most intimate relationship you will ever have is with food.** No? Why? What's the first thing you did when you were born? Breathe? And then? Had milk? Well, do you know that your lungs are actually an off-shoot of your gastrointestinal tract? So even before making provision for you to breathe, Mother Nature made provision for you to eat. Your intestines are supposed to be your first point of contact with the world, in a way your intestines surround you and allow you to interact with both the outside and inside worlds.

Way too often we use food as a means of filling a void that we may be experiencing, to seek love, approval or intimacy, but all this leads to is filling the body with excess fat which reduces its mobility, stability and utility. Ironically, it actually reduces our ability to give and receive love, approval and intimacy. Food, often referred to as dravya in our ancient texts, is meant to heal, strengthen and nourish the body. And the body is meant for a higher purpose, that of achieving the maximum human potential, that of enlightenment.

We have our bodies, just like we have bed sheets, a pair of jeans, etc., but at no point do we *become* the bed sheet or jeans, right? We accept that they are useful for the purpose that we have them for, and understand that we can use them as long as we take care of them and no matter how well we take care of them, one day you will give up the bed sheet.

The food you eat is your way of internalising (and becoming a part of) the universe. So what do you want to internalise? The fresh warmth of 'home-cooked, grown-with-love fruits, veggies, grains, dals, legumes, milk (hey! I am thinking that you are going to buy into my 'farm mother' concept), eaten in peace, digested with calm, absorbed with care, assimilated with responsibility and excreted with sensibility' food? Or the 'well-packaged (low-fat, fibre-enriched, fortified with calcium or some such "eye ball grabber" on the cover), made for the convenience-seeking, gullible buyer, eaten — sorry grabbed — on-the-go, digested with distraction, absorbed minimally, assimilated with stress and excreted with strain' food?

As with all things in life, the choice is totally yours.

Appendices

APPENDIX I
Starting the day right: a comparison of traditional and on-the-go breakfast options

A good beginning is ninety per cent of the weight-loss battle won! So begin your day with a hot, homemade, traditional nashta. You'll see, from the following chart, how a traditional Indian breakfast beats your 'low-calorie' cereal/milk any day. You just need to be smart about varying your breakfast every day so that you expose your body to the maximum number of nutrients on a daily basis.

Most of the homemade breakfast options given can be cooked within fifteen minutes (provided the raw material needed for it is procured and kept ready). It's important to plan your day in advance. Although this requires some time off from your 'busy' schedule, it's an investment that is surely worth it because it is absolutely essential for a fit and toned body — something that adds value to your life and well-being.

These are approximate values for a healthy and happy serving: not too much to make you feel stuffed, not too little that you're left unsatisfied. ☺

Food item	Calories (kcals)	Protein (g)	CHO (g)	Fat (g)	Iron (mg)	Calcium (mg)	Fibre(g)
Aloo Paratha	400	7.6	65	10.1	3.42	38.8	9.2

Nutrient composition: Homemade aloo paratha with ghee is a wholesome meal with a high satiety value, rich in essential fat (ghee). Aloo is a good source of B6 (pyridoxine), vitamin C, potassium, manganese, essential amino acid tryptophan and phytonutrients — carotenoids, flavonoids. It is also a good source of natural dietary fibre, in the adequate amount required (which will not interfere with the absorption of vitamins and minerals).

Spices like ajwain help improve digestion as well as have anti-flatulence properties.

Cosmetic use: Will prevent you from feeling bloated.

Food item	Calories (kcals)	Protein (g)	CHO (g)	Fat (g)	Iron (mg)	Calcium (mg)	Fibre(g)
Idli/ Dosa + Sambhar + Chutney	334	12	54	7	2.09	98.5	10.58

Nutrient composition: Idli + sambhar + chutney is a complete meal with an appropriate balance of carbs, protein, fat, vitamins and minerals. Idli/dosa is a rich source of B12, along with essential fats. Being a cereal-pulse combination, it has all the essential amino acids. Spices like turmeric and mustard add to the nutrient value of this meal. Mustard is rich in selenium and therefore has a strong antioxidant quality. Turmeric, which is a natural colouring and flavouring agent, is also an antiseptic, and has anti-inflammatory and healing properties.

Cosmetic use: For dark circles and puffy eyes.

Food item	Calories (kcals)	Protein (g)	CHO (g)	Fat (g)	Iron (mg)	Calcium (mg)	Fibre(g)
Poha	290	6.45	42.6	9.46	7.1	54.9	6.28

Nutrient composition: Poha is the most common breakfast option, and is an ideal meal in itself. Rice flakes are a good source of iron, and if you squeeze a lemon into it, you will improve on your iron absorption as well. Traditionally peanuts are added to it, which contain MUFA, essential amino acids — tryptophan, B vitamins — niacin, biotin, folate. It is also rich in oleic acid (the essential fat found in olive oil as well) along with high concentrations of antioxidants, especially polyphenols. Spices such as curry leaves and mustard are natural flavouring agents which improve the digestive function by increasing salivary secretion and secretion of digestive juices, improving the function of the small intestine and hence enhancing nutrient absorption.

Cosmetic use: Will get you closer to a flat tummy.

Food item	Calories (kcals)	Protein (g)	CHO (g)	Fat (g)	Iron (mg)	Calcium (mg)	Fibre(g)
Suji halwa	360	1.56	30	20.12	0.26	4.2	1.87

Nutrient composition: Suji halwa is the most loved as well as the most avoided breakfast option ☺. This is the best way to start your day, if you are a sweet lover. The richness of homemade ghee, blended well with semolina and sugar will give you a nutrient-dense meal — all your essential fats, MUFA along with B-complex vitamins. Essential fats will help lubricate your joints, lower your sweet cravings, improve your fat metabolism, reduce your stubborn fat stores, give you a feeling of satiety and will calm your nerves and senses. B-complex vitamins will help improve your carbohydrate metabolism, improve the utilisation of carbs, proteins and fat from your meal. (Even though suji halwa is not high in fibre, the ghee present in it acts as a natural laxative and promotes peristalsis as well.)

Cosmetic use: For soft, smooth and supple skin.

Note: Do not have it every day.

Food item	Calories (kcals)	Protein (g)	CHO (g)	Fat (g)	Iron (mg)	Calcium (mg)	Fibre(g)
Poori bhaji	425	4.6	43.6	25.1	1.95	24.4	5.45

Nutrient composition: Poori bhaji is a traditional breakfast in the east (where it's called luchi aloo), but is considered unhealthy because of its 'high fat' content. Poori bhaji is a wholesome meal which has a good satiety value. It is a good source of vitamins (B-complex and vitamin C), minerals and phytonutrients. Condiments and herbs like cumin seeds, ginger and coriander help improve the palatability, have therapeutic properties and also help improve our metabolism (by aiding digestion). Cumin seeds (jeera) are a good source of iron and manganese. Jeera helps keep our immune system healthy, boosts proper digestion and nutrient assimilation. Ginger is regarded as an excellent carminative (a substance which promotes the elimination of intestinal gas) and intestinal spasmolytic (a substance which relaxes and soothes the intestinal tract), has an anti-inflammatory and anti-carcinogenic action. Coriander has essential oils which have anti-rheumatic and anti-arthritic properties, is an effective diuretic (helps lower high blood pressure) and plays a role in stimulating the digestive juices and peristalsis.

Cosmetic use: Will prevent dandruff and dry skin.

Food item	Calories (kcals)	Protein (g)	CHO (g)	Fat (g)	Iron (mg)	Calcium (mg)	Fibre(g)
Processed commercial cereals with skimmed milk	220	7.9	29.5	8	1.5	180	3.3

Nutrient composition: Processed/commercial cereals with skimmed milk, which is now supposed to be the 'ideal on-the-go' convenience breakfast option is not as healthy compared to your traditional breakfast options.

You don't really feel satisfied with the serving size mentioned on the box (30 g), which leaves you feeling hungrier and makes your sweet cravings shoot up through the day. So even though it is considered a 'low-calorie breakfast', you actually end up eating a SMALL chotu piece of chocolate post-lunch or a pastry post-dinner. This is because when you start your day off with a meal that doesn't give you the kind of satiety and nutrients that you require (after a night of fasting because you are sleeping), you will definitely end up eating much more through the day (your body needs to make up for the calorie deficit). And to top it, all commercial/packaged cereals are loaded with preservatives, artificial colouring and flavouring agents, which not only hamper your nutrient absorption but also compromises the functioning of your digestive tract and strips you off your existing nutrient stores.

Cosmetic use: Complete zero investment of time.

Processed commercial cereal v/s hot homemade breakfast

India has a tradition of hot breakfasts and lunches (as opposed to the Western trend of cold breakfasts and lunches). As Indians we feel more satisfied with a hot, savoury meal rather than a sweetened cold cereal. So even though a hot meal is considered a big luxury in the West, we do not value this privilege of ours in India.

The biggest advantage of eating a hot, cooked breakfast is that it is fresh, homemade, complete with the required nutrients — carbs, proteins, fats, vitamins, macro and micro minerals and many more undiscovered vitamins and minerals.

Homemade nashta does not have artificial colouring or flavouring agents and is preservative free. So nutrient absorption and assimilation from this meal is not compromised. In fact, the natural herbs and spices added to it (which are natural colouring and flavouring agents) will improve your digestion, thereby improving your metabolism through the day. It also satisfies your taste buds and leaves you feeling much more energetic, keeps your blood sugar levels stable and reduces your sweet cravings through the day (absolutely necessary for us — women — to handle PMS, ease out on the pain associated with it, allow our hormones to feel happy and well fed, especially in conditions like thyroid malfunctioning and PCOS).

With processed/commercial cereals, which come with added fibre and vitamins, assimilation is the biggest challenge. This meal is inadequate in terms of the right ratio of carbs, proteins, fats, thus affecting the absorption of vitamins and minerals (since vitamins and minerals will be absorbed and assimilated well only in the presence of carbs, proteins and fat). Also, the type of sugar present in packaged cereals is simple and the ratio of Simple : Complex sugars is usually skewed versus the Simple : Complex sugar ratio in homemade breakfast items.

We need to be much more sensible with our food choices and stay as grounded to our culture and traditional meals rather than just following the Western 'developed or consumerist culture' of 'convenience ready-to-eat meals' which are not just low in calories but also in nutrients! So invest in setting up an efficient kitchen at home, get a well-trained cook if required or learn cooking — even better!

APPENDIX II
Short-term and long-term effects of low-calorie diets

The goal of eating right is to enjoy a higher degree of health and well-being; it is not to restrict the number of calories. An improved nutritional status will help the body let go off unwanted fat stores. A yummy body is a direct output/result of yummy food. We need to understand that if even one of our systems — be it the GI tract, liver or heart — do not function efficiently, it's almost impossible to enjoy good health. It is important for us to value that what food adds to our life goes much beyond the number of calories or serving size. Here are some of the effects of a 'low-calorie' diet.

Meal	Short-term side effects	Long-term side effects
Cereal + low fat milk	It doesn't satisfy your taste buds and leaves you feeling hungry through the day. It lowers your energy levels and so eventually you might just reach out for that piece of chocolate or cake.	The cereal contains preservatives, sodium, additives and emulsifiers which weaken your intestine's ability to absorb and assimilate nutrients, leading to nutrient deficiencies and poor nutrient stores. The milk is stripped off the essential fats which actually help burn stubborn fat, and also lubricate your bones and joints. Eventually you will develop long-term deficiencies.

Meal	Short-term side effects	Long-term side effects
Commercial and packaged juices	The juice is nothing but coloured water that is not really providing your body with any nutrients because as soon as a fruit/vegetable is cut and exposed to the environment, it starts losing its nutrients as well.	Fruits and veggies are meant to be chewed, not drunk. Fruits and veggies are loaded with antioxidants, so stripping the fruit/veggie off its fibre and nutrients adds to your nutrient deficiencies and lowers your body's ability to cope with any kind of stress. So rather than just popping antioxidants, have your whole fruit and keep it fresh and seasonal.
Steamed veggies + fibre-added roti	Steamed veggies will actually make you feel sick: you won't feel like eating a good portion because it tastes so bland! The fibre-added roti will worsen the situation and you will end up eating only a small portion of this meal, and feel that you have learnt not to overeat. But you aren't getting any nourishment out of this meal, the sole reason being you didn't really enjoy what you were eating.	The fibre added to the roti is only going to add to your body's woes of absorbing nutrients, especially calcium and iron. Though you are taking enough fibre, you have no fat source to lubricate it, so you are definitely going to end up feeling constipated and bloated and will end up taking a laxative.
Retricted diets comprising mostly fruits like orange/sweet lime	The body needs proper carbs, protein and fat to assimilate anything from the fruit, so you need to have a good nutritional status if you wish to get the maximum benefits out of a fruit. If you are on a low-calorie diet, your nutrient assimilation from the fruit is going to be absolutely NIL (because vitamins and minerals are absorbed only if the diet provides adequate carbs, protein and fats).	We try to stick to 'low-calorie' fruits like orange, sweet lime and avoid seasonal fruits like mango, seetaphal, strawberries, chickoo thinking that they are 'high in sugar' and 'fattening'. It is absolutely necessary to eat seasonal fruits because nature produces them at a time when their nutrients are peaking and you can get the maximum nutrient absorption and assimilation. Avoid going against nature — else nature will go against you ☺.

Meal	Short-term side effects	Long-term side effects
Dry bhel or kurmura	It's like a punishment to your body and mainly your palate, so the enzymes won't be secreted and optimum digestion will not take place, leaving you feeling bloated (you will just be burping and farting all the time ☺).	Eating dry bhel is like watching Salman Khan with his shirt on ;). You get absolutely no nutrients out of this meal; even if there are any nutrients present, absorption and assimilation is absolutely zero. So you are just having a low-calorie meal that is low in nutrients as well. Such meals will aggravate your nutrient deficiencies, keeping you irritable through the day, and increase your risk to fractures and joint pains. Instead, eat your bhel with the date and coriander chutney which will improve the nutrient to calorie ratio of your meal.
Soup and salad: the 'classic' meal ☺	This is the most common dinner option — the 'killer' combination. The salad has been cut god knows when and if you add low-fat dressing to it you are giving your body its daily quota of preservatives and salt as well! The veggies in the soup have been cut, mashed, blended, strained and boiled like there's no tomorrow, ensuring that there are no nutrients left at all. Even though you feel full after this meal, it may leave you reaching out for a coffee or pastry later — a complete diet disaster.	By restricting your intake of complete meals, you don't really expose your body to different food groups because your focus is just 'low-calories'. You're not considering the aspect of low nutrients that comes with this kind of diet. In the long run, this nutritionally underpowered status will take you nowhere except add to your vitamin and mineral deficiencies — the most common being calcium, vitamins B12 and D3 (disaster for thyroid and PCOS). So although you will surely 'lose weight', you will also lose your charm, state of mind, energy levels and sleep! Please be sensible about WHAT you are eating and not how many calories you are consuming.

Word of caution: The process of making packaged juices actually strips the fruits of all the nutrients. There is absolutely no packaged juice which is preservative-free. To make the juice, first a concentrate is prepared — the process involves exposing the fruit pulp to high temperatures and a lot of churning/grinding, which will surely not keep any of the vitamins intact.

Packaged cereals and fruit juices are commonly sold with misleading labels, such as '100% fresh' (any food which has added preservatives can never be fresh), 'preservative-free' (which is impossible considering their long shelf life), 'added fibre and fortified with iron/ calcium' (something which cannot be absorbed by your body; in fact, excess artificial fibre will interfere with the absorption of nutrients, especially calcium and iron).

APPENDIX III

Foods considered healthy ... and why they're not

	Food item considered healthy	Why it's considered healthy ...	And why it's not
1	Multi-grain or bran attas vs wheat, jowar, bajra, ragi, atta	Because of the high fibre content	Excess fibre binds with calcium and minerals and so hampers absorption. Also, the many grains mixed in the multigrain atta leads to poor absorption of nutrients since they compete for absorption in our body. In the bargain, you end up absorbing much less than what is available.
2	Baked chips vs fried chips	Because it is considered to be a low-calorie, low-fat food	The process of baking needs some form of fat (shortening agents) and preservatives (baking soda) which are added at the time of baking. Also, since it is considered to be healthy, you will definitely end up overeating as compared to fried chips.
3	Multi-grain biscuits over regular/cream biscuits	Considered to high fibre biscuits which make you feel less hungry	Since they are loaded with preservatives and fat (which is needed for the baking process), it drains your body of all the nutrients because it's a Herculean task for your body to digest such highly processed foods. Also, since you consider it to be healthy, you will tend to overeat. I prefer regular or cream biscuits — at least you are aware that you are consuming a high-fat, high-sugar product and will exercise caution. Moreover they taste better than the 'fibre enriched' variety.
4	Low-fat, low-cholesterol butter vs regular butter/ghee	Because it is considered to be low in fat	It contains less saturated fat but contains trans fat which impairs fat metabolism, whereas the essential fats in homemade ghee/butter actually improve fat metabolism.
5	Sukha bhel vs regular bhel	Because the sweet chutney in regular bhel contains sugar and dates which are high in calories	The chutney actually makes regular bhel more nutrient-dense and palatable. And trust me, it adds negligible calories to your bhel.

6	Low-fat cheese vs regular fat cheese	Because it is considered to be low-fat, thus healthy	Because low-fat cheese is processed to the extent that it gets stripped of all its nutrients (calcium, protein) and is also low in essential fatty acid, CLA, which is necessary to improve fat metabolism.
7	Dry fruits (almonds) vs peanuts	Considered to be good sources of vitamins, especially vitamin E	It is healthy when eaten in the right quantity and at the right time. It is definitely not something you should be munching on because it is high in fat as well. So if you snack on it thinking it is 'healthy', you may end up overeating. Just because it's more expensive than peanuts doesn't make it better. So allow your body to be exposed to the goodness of the humble channa and singdana too.
8	Sweeteners/ brown sugar vs regular white sugar	Considered to be low in calories	Since it is considered to be low in calories, you tend to take it in larger quantities. Sweeteners also contain chemicals which affects brain functioning (irreversible brain damage, epileptic seizures), leads to hormonal imbalances, insulin insensitivity, loss of hair and many more side effects.
9	Soups and salads vs a complete meal (roti + sabzi + dal)	Considered healthy because of its very low caloric content	Food is not limited to only numbers. Rather than calories, it is more important to see what nutrients the food is giving you. Because soup has been blended and overcooked, it loses all its nutrient value, so it is as good as having coloured water. Salads are rich in vitamins and minerals and a good source of fibre, but absorbed best only if it is eaten with a balanced/ complete meal.
10	Fruit juices vs whole fruit	Considered to be skin-friendly and responsible for that glowing skin	When cut, fruits are exposed to sunlight and start losing their vitamins and minerals, so by the time you make them into juice and have it, you have almost deprived your body of all the nutrients the fruit has. Also, because you would need a larger portion of fruits to make a fruit juice compared to what you would eat, it will cause a spike in your blood sugar.

| 11 | Popcorn vs makhana | Popcorn is considered the ultimate low-cal snack | Come on, since when did butter with salt become a low-cal snack? Ever tried makhana after roasting it in a kadhai with ghee, salt and pepper? It's rich in nutrients, great to taste and crisp to the core. What's more? It even looks better than popcorn. Saif, a self-confessed popcorn addict, has converted to makhana. Checked out how he's looking? |

Appendix IV

Is your body talking to you? Nutrition deficiencies and how to combat them

Oh no!	What is it?	Are you doing this?	You know what...	Do this instead...
Water retention	• Protein deficiency	• Eating 'low-calorie'/'low-fat' biscuits, 'diet snacks' (low-calorie diet)?	By not providing your body with the desired amount of carbs, proteins, fats, your body's nourishment status is being compromised. A low-carb diet will actually deplete your protein stores, because proteins will need to do the function of carbs in your body and at the same time its own functions as well. Low protein levels will lead to edema (water retention) — your body cells release water into your tissues instead of eliminating it the natural way.	• Eat fresh wholesome meals with the right balance of carbs, protein and fat.
	• Sodium and potassium electrolyte imbalance	• Eating chips, bakery products and packaged foods (processed foods with excess sodium)?	The excess sodium in processed foods will disturb the electrolyte balance in your body. Sodium holds on to water, therefore this will lead to water retention.	• Eat freshly cooked meals and restrict your intake of processed foods to once a week.
	• Dehydration	• Consuming low calorie/aerated drinks, excess tea, coffee?	All these beverages are dehydrating, leading to water storage in the body. (Only when your body does not get adequate water does it need to store water.)	• Drink enough water instead. To let your body get rid of the excess water stores, keep your body hydrated at all times.

Oh no!	What is it?	Are you doing this?	You know what...	Do this instead...
Breakouts	• Lack of vitamins A, C and E, chromium and zinc (mainly antioxidants)	• Having canned juices, biscuits, pastries loaded with sugar?	The excess sugar in the canned juices/beverages, biscuits will interfere with the absorption of certain minerals, leading to deficiency of these vitamins and minerals in the body.	Eat whole fresh fruits and vegetables so that your body gets the maximum nutrients from these. (Fruits and veggies lose their nutrients the longer they are left cut, with exposure to light and heat.)
	• Dehydration	• Eating out at restaurants regularly?	Alcohol completely washes away all the vitamin B stores and friendly bacteria from the digestive tract, thereby reducing the efficiency of the digestive system.	Eat fresh, wholesome meals prepared at home, as the nutrient value of these foods is much higher than processed foods.
		• Drinking alcohol often?		Drink more water instead. Water will help wash out all the toxins from your system, improve circulation and keep your cells well hydrated.

Oh no!	What is it?	Are you doing this?	You know what...	Do this instead...
Hair loss, split ends and dandruff	• Protein deficiency • Essential fatty acid deficiency, especially Omega-3 • Vitamin B6, B12 and folic acid deficiency • Zinc deficiency	• Having dry rotis without ghee, cooking vegetables in extra refined oils, having fat-free milk? • Eliminating carbs post lunch, having a 'low carb' diet? • Regularly taking steroids/contraceptives/birth control pills? • Taking laxatives and having bingeing-purging episodes.	Deficiency in protein, essential fat and zinc (caused by low-calorie/low-carb diets, medication) prevent healthy hair growth and makes the hair look dull, frizzy, dry.	For healthy lustrous hair, you need to provide your body with adequate protein (for long and strong hair and to prevent hair fall), essential fat (for the lustre and smoothness), zinc (helps in rebuilding hair and prevent hair loss), vitamins B6 and B12 and folic acid (enables hair growth by helping to provide a constant supply of blood and oxygen to the hair follicles). So rather than just banking on those hair treatment products, make sure you meet your body's requirements of all the above nutrients.
Brittle nails and white spots on nails	• Protein, calcium, zinc deficiency	• Following/followed all possible starvation and fad diets to achieve that figure/number on the weighing scale? • Drinking a lot of black tea/juices/diet colas through the day?	Though you are trying to restrict the intake of calories in the day, you are also compromising on your body's nutrient requirements and nutrient stores. In fact, starvation actually depletes your body's stores of muscle protein, calcium (to maintain the optimum pH in your body) and micominerals — especially zinc — which leads to slow growth and loss of appetite, further aggravating the starvation state.	By now we know that protein has a wide cosmetic function in our body. To ensure that the protein function is not compromised on — so that the protein is used for the right purpose by our body — we need to ensure adequate carb intake on a regular basis (calcium and zinc also require adequate protein for absorption). So make sure you are eating your carbs along with protein in every meal.

Oh no!	What is it?	Are you doing this?	You know what...	Do this instead...
Scaled lips	• Deficiency of vitamin B2, niacin and B6	• Taking medication/drugs/ birth control pills or painkillers or a sedative every day? • On a restricted diet?	All these drugs will strip your system of its B vitamin stores.	Avoid long-term use of these medications/drugs. Switch to a healthier eating pattern and expose your body to different food groups to get the maximum nutrient exposure. Limit your intake of processed foods.
Dry skin and lips	• Deficiency of essential fat • Deficiency of biotin	• Having low fat milk, limiting oil usage to extra virgin olive oil/'heart-healthy' oils/avoiding ghee, eating steamed veggies/ boiled veggies without tadka?	Without an adequate amount of fat (essential fat) in the diet, our skin loses its moisture and therefore turns dry.	Drink your milk and nariyal pani with the malai; do not exclude any form of essential fat from your diet. This is because, for your body to absorb vitamins and minerals, it needs a baseline diet adequate in essential fats (along with carbs and protein). These fats are required in order to keep the skin well hydrated, moist, smooth and supple.
Puffiness below eyes, eye bags and dark circles	• Vitamin K, B12, B6 and iron deficiency	• Are you on anti-hypertensives (BP control drugs), consuming processed and packaged foods (excess salt), smoking regularly?	Excess dietary salt, smoking and anti-hypertensives cause blood vessels under the eyes to dilate and get engorged, which can contribute to dark circles and puffiness.	Do not suppress your appetite by smoking. Instead, eat fresh wholesome foods which will improve overall blood circulation and blood flow.

Oh no!	What is it?	Are you doing this?	You know what…	Do this instead…
One tooth turning yellow	Vitamin C and calcium deficiency	• Leaving long gaps between your meals?	Long gaps between meals lead to increased acid secretion in the body, which affects the body's calcium stores. The teeth are immediately affected.	Have regular, frequent meals through the day. Instead of eating 2-3 large meals a day, eat at regular intervals in order to maintain the right pH balance in the stomach and prevent acidity.
		• Having a lot of carbonated beverages, soft drinks, coffee, tea?	Carbonated beverages, coffee and tea have adverse effects on bone mineral density (BMD) because they lower calcium and vitamin C absorption which are vital to maintain good dental health.	Restrict your intake of tea/coffee to a maximum of 2 cups a day and carbonated beverages to not more than once a week.
Pigmentation and patchy skin	Deficiency of iron, B12, calcium and vitamins D3, A and E	• Consuming laxatives on a regular basis? • Using an excess of sunscreens and sun blocks?	The excess fibre/laxative actually hampers the absorption of vitamins and minerals — especially calcium and iron — by binding to it and excreting it through faeces.	Make sure you are eating well, consuming enough carbs to enable the absorption of B12 and incorporating essential fat to enable absorption of vitamin A and E (fat-soluble vitamins). Also, make sure you are waking up close to sunrise — or at least between 6-8 a.m. — to ensure enough exposure to sunlight and allow maximum vitamin D3 absorption. Your body can absorb the maximum nutrients from what you eat at this time as well.

348 ∞ *Rujuta Diwekar*

Appendix V

More sample diets and activity recalls

Sabiha Khan is a young, chirpy twenty-five-year-old IT consultant.

She studied at IIT Delhi and had lived there for most of her student life till she shifted to Chandigarh for work (it's also where her parents live).

She has her mother's taste in food — she loves her parathas, lassi and chole bhature.

In school, she was interested in sports and would actively participate in all sports tournaments, excelling in basketball and volleyball.

She wanted to make a career in IT, so had to give up on sports, since her course required competitive examinations and a lot of stress! (Sounds familiar?) This was the time when she developed PCOS and acne (which she was ashamed of). Since then she has been on contraceptive pills (that's what she was prescribed for PCOD and acne).

She has done some crash diets in her struggle to remain 'fit', as well as 'detox' diets, one-day protein, one-day carb diets, etc.

She loves her work and is a thorough workaholic, but now she has decided to be as committed towards her health and body. She feels what she did in the past was not the right thing for her body and now wants to focus on a healthier lifestyle, improve her fitness levels and get back to what she was in her school days.

Three-day diet recall

Time	Food/Drink	Activity Recall	Workout
Day 1			
5.30 – 5.45 a.m.	2 glasses of water	Woke up and freshened up	
5.45 a.m.	6 pieces of litchis + 2 glasses of warm water		
6.15 – 7.00 a.m.			Walked to the park, jogged and stretched there

7.30 a.m.	1 glass milk with Bournvita	Chatted with friends at the park, got back home and freshened up	
7.30 – 8.30 a.m.		Showered, got ready	
8.30 a.m.	1 ghiya-stuffed paratha (½ tsp oil) 1 glass water 1 cup chole		
9.00 a.m.		Drove to work	
9.30 a.m.	1 glass water		
9.20 – 11.00 a.m.		Worked at my desk	
11.00 a.m.	1 roti ½ katori chole sabzi		
11.15 a.m. – 3.30 p.m.		Worked	
3.30 p.m.	1 cup noodles (Maggi)		
3.30 - 5.00 p.m.	3-4 glasses water		
3.45 – 5.00 p.m.		Worked	
5.00 p.m.		Left office, drove to a nearby restaurant to meet up with a friend	
5.30 p.m.	½ veg and cheese lasagna 1 glass masala cola		
6.00 – 6.30 p.m.		Went to the temple	
6.30 p.m.		Went home	
6.30 – 8.00 p.m.	2 glasses of water	Watched TV	
8.30 p.m.	1 roti, 1 cup bean sabzi, 2 glasses of water		

| 8.45 – 10.30 p.m. | | Chatted with parents | |
| 11.00 p.m. | | Slept | |

Day 2			
5.30 – 5.45 a.m.	2 glasses of water	Woke up, freshened up	
5.45 a.m.	1 mango		
6.15 – 7.00 a.m.			Walked to the park, did jogging and stretching there
7.20 a.m.	1 glass milk with Bournvita	Chatted with friends at the park and then got back home	
7.30 – 8.30 a.m.		Showered, got ready	
8.45 a.m.	1 ghiya stuffed paratha + 1 glass water		
9.15 a.m. – 12 p.m.		Drove to office and worked	
12.15 p.m.	½ chocolate, 1 roti, 1 cup arhar dal, ½ cup mushroom		
12.45 – 3.00 p.m.	3 glasses of water	Worked	
3.00 p.m.		Took a break, went for a stroll in office	
3.15 – 5.15 p.m.	Handful of channa + 4 glasses of water	Worked	
5.30 p.m.		Got back home	
6.00 – 8.00 p.m.		Watched TV, chatted with mom and dad	
8.00 p.m.	1½ cup rice, 1 cup arhar dal, ½ cup bhindi, 1 glass sweet lassi		
11.00 p.m.		Slept	

Day 3 (Holiday)			
6 a.m.		Woke up, freshened up	
6.30 a.m.	1 glass milk with Bournvita		
6.45 – 8.30 a.m.		Read newspaper, chatted with parents	
8.30 a.m.	1½ cup poha, 1 glass salted lassi		
9.00 – 11.00 a.m.	1 glass water	Showered, did puja, chatted with parents	
11.00 a.m. – 1.30 p.m.		Went shopping	
1.45 p.m.	1½ cup rice, 1 cup rajma, 1 glass fresh lime water		
3.00 p.m.	Handful of channa		
4.00 – 6.30 p.m.		Went for movie	
7.00 p.m.	1 glass of water		
8.30 p.m.	2 roti, 1 cup rajma, 1 piece coconut barfi		
9.45 p.m.		Slept	

Evaluation of the recall

Sabiha just needed to eat right and exercise regularly (she is an early riser and goes to bed at a regular time, which made my work simpler ☺). Though her PCOD was under control, she wanted to get rid of her acne.

As we all know by now, whenever your body is deprived of the right nutrients — especially during earlier adulthood (between eighteen and twenty-two, which is actually a growing stage for girls, where their ovaries mature and their body shape changes into a more feminine one) — the body's cells remain deprived of much-needed nutrients, leading to hormonal imbalances causing ovaries to become overworked and stressed out, finally arising as PCOS.

Sabiha was always stressed during her college years because she wanted to excel in what she was doing, even at the cost of her health and diet. She had opted for crash diets that put her body through additional stress. A combination of mental and physical stress (very common) is a well known cause of PCOS.

Since Sabiha had been a sports person in her school days, she was at least protected from a full-blown hormonal imbalance that can lead to many more disorders such as thyroid and diabetes.

Now, at work, she had the flexibility to leave early or come late, and she loved her job too, so her level of stress was not as much as it was in her earlier years. But what you are today is always a reflection of what you have done when you were fifteen, eighteen, twenty, and Sabiha had to bear the brunt of it too.

Though her condition had improved (she believes it all happened only after reading the book ☺), she wanted to get back to her earlier fitness levels and build good nutrient stores, enough to support her thirties, forties, fifties and sixties!

Modifications
Sabiha simply needs to clean up her diet and eat wholesome nutritious meals to support her ovaries. She also needs to exercise regularly (challenging her fitness levels).

The best part is that she has always had a lot of family support throughout (which did help lower her stress levels — especially when she had to shift from Delhi to Chandigarh for her job).

She can modify her diet as follows:

Meal 1 (5.45 a.m.): Banana/fresh seasonal fruit (She loves seasonal fruits — especially mangoes)

Meal 2 (7.30 a.m.), post workout, within 10 mins: Protein shake: 1 scoop in water + banana

Meal 3 (8.30 – 8.45 a.m.): Freshly cooked homemade seviyan upma/paratha with veggies + coriander chutney (her traditional breakfast)

Meal 4 (10.30 a.m.): Fruit yogurt/lassi salted (she prefers something sweet or salty — easy to carry to work)

Meal 5 (12.00 p.m.): Roti/rice + sabzi + dal (1 tsp homemade ghee; could carry lunch from home or mother could send a dabba, her office being fifteen minutes away from work)

Meal 6 (2.00 p.m.): Roasted channa

Meal 7 (4.00 p.m.): Cheese chilly toast (needed a good wholesome meal at this time, but also something convenient at work)

Meal 8 (6.00 p.m.): Fresh fruit

Meal 9 (7.00 p.m.) Roti/rice + sabzi + dal (enjoy a freshly cooked dinner)

Meal 10 (9.00 p.m.): Protein shake: ½ scoop in milk (to ensure good overnight recovery)

She was also advised to take essential fats — Omega-3 and 6 along with B12, zinc, chromium with antioxidants — mainly to improve her hormonal functioning, sensitising her cells to absorb much more nutrients and lowering her fat stores, by providing essential fats (with MUFA as well)

Once Sabiha started off, there was no looking back. She improved every week and in fact in the first week itself she felt she was a different person altogether. She ate her meals exactly on time and loved it. She would look forward to all her meals, would sleep exactly on time and wake up in time to go for her morning workouts.

Her sweet cravings had become minimal, she felt energetic as never before (not even during her school days), she was losing inches and looking much leaner than before.

Her father, who is a doctor, now feels for the very first time that she is on the right track and has made the right choice of improving her health rather than just focusing on weight loss.

Being in the younger age group and having a background in sports, her body had the muscle memory, which was an added boost and gave her very good results.

She is currently enjoying her courtship (yes, she got engaged during her programme) and is loving all the compliments she gets from her fiancé — she feels she is the perfect shape she had never even dreamt of!

Elizabeth is a twenty-nine-year-old customer service officer.

Her work pattern is very stressful and she shuttles between morning and night shifts. She tends to make incorrect food choices because of stress at work. She feels very lethargic in the morning when she wakes up as well as through the day, even after she sleeps well.

She suffers from borderline osteopenia, which she discovered after a DXA scan. Until then she felt that the back pain and leg pain was only because of standing so much and wearing heels.

This is how Elizabeth describes her job: 'I work as an officer, wherein I am in charge of at least thirty-five flights per day, so I've got to monitor every movement, need to closely monitor full flights and excessively delayed flights which takes a lot of my energy which I hardly have. The job is not creative, but it involves a lot of convincing, talking, arguing, handling staff, getting fired and firing back!'

She lives with her father and has to do all the household work by herself. She doesn't eat freshly-prepared meals, and cooks food only once a day, which lasts till the next day afternoon. Her 'holiday' comprises working at home and running errands.

Three-day diet recall

Day 1			
Time	Food/Drink	Activity Recall	Workout
3.15 a.m.		Woke up and got ready	
4.00 a.m.	1 orange, 4 walnuts, ¼ cup milk, 1 small til laddoo and 1 tab of B-complex		

4.20 a.m.		The pick-up arrived, went by car to work	
5.00 – 7.30 a.m.		At work desk, monitoring my flights, very stressed already talking and arguing with passengers. After this, went to the canteen	
8.00 a.m.	White bread sandwich (3 layers), spread with green chutney and egg (boiled) 2 sips of water 1 cup coffee (cutting types)		
8.45 a.m.		Back at counter, doing the same job	
10.30 a.m.	Got little time, hence had 1 sip of water		
11.00 a.m. – 12.00 p.m.		Updated reports at work	
12.30 p.m.	2 pieces of chikki (groundnut) and had 2 khakara	Left work. On the way to the coach, picked up chikki and khakhra	
12.45 p.m.		Got on to the coach, lots of traffic every day	
1.30 p.m.		Reached home, had a shower	
2.00 p.m.	½ cup of Kissan orange squash		
2.15 p.m.	3 small spoons of rice, pork curry and red, yellow capsicum peppers 2 sips of water	Watched TV	
3.00 – 6.30 p.m.		Slept. Got up feeling very drained and tired. Had a large bottle of water	

Time	Food	Activity	
6.35 p.m.	Coffee and 3-4 chocolate wafer sticks (cylindrical thin)	.	,
7.45 – 8.45 p.m.			Went for a walk
9.07 p.m.		Reached home and had a shower	
9.25 p.m.	1 katori rice, fish curry (2 pieces only), 3 sips of water. Dinner over by 9.44 p.m.		
9.55 p.m.	1 mango		
10.30 p.m.	¼ cup warm milk, with a pinch of haldi		
10.50 p.m.		In bed	
Day 2			
3.15 a.m.		Woke up and got ready	
4.00 a.m.	1 orange, 4 walnuts, ¼ cup milk, 1 small til laddoo and 1 tab of B-complex		
4.20 a.m.		The pick-up arrived. Went by car to work	
5.00 – 7.30 a.m.		Monitoring flights at work	
7.45 a.m.		Walked to canteen	
8.00 a.m.	White bread sandwich (3 layers), spread with green chutney and egg (boiled) 2 sips of water 1 cup coffee (cutting types)		
8.30 a.m.		Came back to counter and did a bit of floor supervision	
10 a.m.	A few sips of water		

10.53 a.m.	2 handfuls of brown channa		
11 a.m.		Started updating reports	
12.09 p.m.		Head was paining, had coffee, cutting	
12.20 p.m.	Soya chaklis (8-9 small pieces)		
1.00 – 1.30 p.m.		Today there was a briefing to be conducted for all staff. Went home by rickshaw, reached at 2.18 p.m. Had a shower	
2.38 p.m.	Brown channa curry, rice, coconut base curry, lunch over by 2.52 p.m.	Watched TV	
2.52 – 3.25 p.m.	Ate 1 choco wafer stick 3.00 p.m. Ate another choco wafer stick 3.25 p.m. Ate 6 choco wafer sticks	Watched TV then started preparing dinner	
3.45 – 6.00 p.m.		Slept	
6.35 p.m.	Coffee		
6.42 p.m.	A few sips of water		
7.00 – 8.00 p.m.			Yoga class
8.17 p.m.	A few sips of Kissan orange squash		
8.40 p.m.		Went out with friends	
9.45 p.m.	Papa Jones chicken barbeque pizza and garlic bread (3 pieces each)	Walked from restaurant to the house. Reached home at 10.19 p.m. Watched TV	
11.35 p.m.		In bed	

Day 3 (Holiday)			
9.20 a.m.		Woke up, brushed	
9.30 a.m.	Had a banana		
9.50 a.m.	1 cup tea, 4 slices of bread, toasted		
10.40 a.m.		Did some dusting around the house	
11 a.m.	Had a few sips of water	Lay down on the bed, just lazing	
11.52 a.m.		Went down to get something photocopied. Walked back home	
12.45 p.m.	1 slab (cylindrical) of malai kulfi		
1.10 p.m.	Rice, shark fish curry 3 pieces, little paneer curry, red peppers A few sips of water with lunch		
1.30 – 2.30 p.m.		Sat at the computer	
2.45 – 6.00 p.m.		Napped	
6.05 p.m.	Coffee		
6.15 p.m.	1 choco wafer stick		
6.25 p.m.		Ironed my uniform	
6.35 p.m.	1 mango		
7.45 p.m.		Showered	
8.35 p.m.	Rice, moong curry, 4 fish nuggets, yellow and red peppers. 8.59 p.m. dinner over.		
9.45 p.m.	¼ cup warm milk, with a pinch of haldi		
9.50 p.m.		Again sat at the computer	
10.20 p.m.		In bed	

Evaluation of the recall

Elizabeth believes she has put on weight and is low on energy levels because of her stressful work and wrong eating habits. She is trying her best to eat healthy, but falls prey to sweet cravings and convenience foods. (This recall is the diet she started after reading *Don't Lose Your Mind, Lose Your Weight*. One can only imagine her original diet!)

When your body is subjected to any kind of stress, mental or physical (which the body can't distinguish between), it releases stress hormones to help your body cope. At such times, your body's nutrient requirements increase and if they are not met, your body starts storing fat. So it is very important to have a stress-free environment in your body, to allow maximum absorption of nutrients.

Elizabeth's body is constantly subjected to stress because she has to cope with her day and night shifts (which makes the body work against it's natural biological clock and creates a stressful environment), monitor flights, deal with clients which involves a lot of shouting and being shouted at (never an easy task)! She also has her responsibilities at home which involve household chores like dusting, ironing, cooking and grocery shopping, which leaves very little time for herself.

After reading *Don't Lose Your Mind, Lose Your Weight,* she decided to at least begin with some form of exercise, so she took up yoga which made her feel balanced.

She sleeps late and barely sleeps well, which makes her feel dull and lethargic when she wakes up in the morning.

Modifications

Elizabeth needs to eat well so that her body has the right nutrients which will help improve her energy levels so she can deal with routine activities at work and home much more efficiently.

She should eat more often and exercise at least three times a week to improve her energy and fitness levels. She needs to sleep early, by 10.30 p.m. latest, since she also starts her day early. This will allow her body to recover well.

Once she makes simple changes like eating right and at regular intervals, exercising regularly and sleeping on time, she will feel much more energetic, fitter, calmer, be more attentive and will be better able to cope with stressful situations at work.

It would be advisable for her to start with weight-training, as she will improve her body's bone mineral density and lean body mass, which will improve her body composition and lower her fat stores. This will also work at strengthening her leg and back muscles to cope with standing and heels (part of the uniform).

She can modify her diet as follows:

Meal 1 (3.15 a.m.): Protein shake (best way to start her day since she needs a lot of recovery)

Meal 2 (5 a.m.): Banana/fresh seasonal fruit (easy to eat and carry to work)

Meal 3 (7 a.m.): Slice of cheese (easy to carry and will satisfy her taste buds as well ☺)

Meal 4 (9 a.m.): 1 slice of bread with chutney + veggies (can pack it at home and carry it along, does not get messy)

Meal 5 (11 a.m.): Soy milk, any flavour (easily available, can stock it in her office or buy it in the office canteen)

Meal 6 (1 p.m.): A handful of peanuts/channa (store at work/carry in her bag)

Meal 7 (3 p.m.): Rice + veg curry (at home)

Meal 8 (5 p.m.): 2 egg whites with veggies + whole wheat toast (easy to cook, at home)

Meal 9 (7 p.m. or post yoga): 1 chapatti + sabzi or sabzi + bowl of dal (have an early dinner at home, so that she can sleep by 10 p.m.

She was advised to take a whey protein supplement, vitamin C and E (antioxidants), B-complex vitamins and calcium. (The whey protein would ensure a good recovery, the other vitamins would help take care of her nutritional deficiencies which would improve her overall nutritional status and help her function more efficiently at work.)

Elizabeth modified her eating pattern as given and it was suggested that she not exercise for the first two weeks, and instead focus on eating right and sleeping on time, as recovery was the main issue. Exercise was introduced only after ensuring that she had reached optimum nutrient status and was sleeping well.

She was also advised to cut down on non-vegetarian food (once or twice a week) and switch to leaner meats. (Non-vegetarian food is tougher to digest and therefore requires more blood flow to be directed to the digestive system to help break it down. But while she was at work, she required a greater blood flow to her brain to keep her more attentive and alert.)

Within a week, she was feeling much more energetic, she was not at all fatigued and she almost started feeling as though her job was not really as stressful as she thought it was! All this was because she was now armed mentally and physically to cope with stressful environments.

About eight weeks later, when she checked her body fat percentage, it was down by almost 2.5 per cent! Another few weeks down the line, she started feeling more toned and her clothes started feeling looser. She had lost a few inches, looked fresher and felt more energetic than she had ever before, and thinks that work shifts are no big deal at all now. She had now started feeling as responsible for herself as she did towards her job.

Priya Lalwani is a thirty-one-year old housewife with two children.

She was married at a very young age (about twenty), and by twenty-one had had the first of her two children, her daughter. Ever since then she has been caught up with her responsibilities at home and cannot see beyond her household work and her kids. Her life revolves around looking after her kids, cooking, shopping for the house, cleaning her house and so on. By the time she is half way through her day, she is exhausted. (Even after an eight-hour sleep at night, she never feels fresh on waking up.)

She had always wanted to work and start a business of her own, but because she is so involved with these responsibilities, she has not managed to do it all these years.

She also feels that, since she got married early, she missed out on having fun with her friends (like going for a girl's night out or bachelorette parties) because she needed to take care of her kids (whom she hadn't planned on having so early).

Now, finally, the one thing that she wants to do for herself is lose weight and look 'thin', so she has decided to get on to a diet programme.

Three-day diet recall

Time	Food/ Drink	Activity Recall	Workout
Day 1			
7.00 a.m.		Wake up, freshened up, showered	
7.15 a.m.	1 cup tea + 8 almonds (had this while working in the kitchen)		

Time	Food	Activity	Exercise
7.30 – 9.30 a.m.		Started preparing husband's tiffin, cleaned my room and children's room; got my son ready	
9.30 a.m.	4 glasses of water	Made my son study for exams	
10.30 a.m.	2 glasses of buttermilk, 2 open toasted sandwiches		
11.30 a.m.	1 piece chikki		
1.15 p.m.	2 jowar rotis, ½ aloo paratha, ½ cup curd, ½ cup dal and ½ cup rice	After lunch went to have fruits and snacks at Breach Candy	
3.00 – 4.00 p.m.		Made my son and daughter study and talked to my architect	
4.00 p.m.		Made tea for myself and others	
4.15 p.m.	Tea + 2 cream crackers	Preparations for dinner	
5.30 p.m.			Went to the gym for one hour
7.30 p.m.	1 cup papaya + soup	Took a shower and did a few things in the kitchen	
8.30 p.m.	1 pizza without cheese	Sat with the kids to make them study	
9.00 p.m.		Watched TV	
11.00 p.m.		Went to sleep	
Day 2			
7.30 a.m.	Tea and 8 almonds	Showered	
8.00 – 10.30 a.m.		Did all household-related work; packed children's tiffin, cleaned my room and put clothes in the cupboard	
10.30 a.m.	2 open toast sandwiches + 2 glasses buttermilk		
11.00 a.m. – 12.00 p.m.			Went to gym

1.15 p.m.	1 pizza + 1 cup curd		
2.00 – 3.00 p.m.		Made the kids study	
3.00 p.m.	1 piece chocolate	Prepared milk for kids and then took a nap	
4.00 p.m.		Prepared tea for kids tuition teacher and myself	
4.15 p.m.	1 cup tea + 2 cream crackers		
5.00 p.m.		Went out shopping while children were having tuition, came home and prepared dinner	
7.30 p.m.	1 bowl papaya + bowl of soup	Sat with guests and then went for shower	
8.45 p.m.	2 chapattis + aloo veg + curd + 2 spoons khichdi		
9.00 p.m.		Made my son study and watched TV	
11.00 p.m.		Went to sleep	
Day 3 (Holiday)			
8.00 a.m.	1 cup tea + almonds	Read newspaper, went for bath, did kitchen work and made son study	
9.30 a.m.	Green tea + fruit		
10.30 a.m.	1 idli + 2 slices of toast + 2 glasses buttermilk		
1.00 p.m.	2 jowar rotis + veg + curd + fried papad		
2.00 – 3.00 p.m.		Made the kids study	
4.00 p.m.	Tea + 2 cream crackers		
6.30 p.m.	Soup + papaya	Chatted with husband	
8.00 p.m.	Out for dinner – Chinese		
11.30 p.m.		Went to sleep	

Evaluation of the recall

As you can see from her recall, Priya starts her day early and has a long day from then on. As soon as she wakes up, she heads to the kitchen, makes herself a cup of tea and has it with a few almonds while she is cooking. (No time to even sit and enjoy her morning tea!)

After that she is constantly running behind her kids — getting them ready for school, packing their dabbas (and also her husband's), making them study, giving them snacks and milk when they come home, cleaning their messy rooms, and so on.

While they are taking tuition, she utilises this time to either go shopping or go for a work out. Priya barely does anything for herself the entire day.

She feels that though she is 'just a housewife' by profession, she is actually multitasking the entire day and doing the job of a maid, cook, cleaner and accountant! She is just so tired at the end of the day, that she can barely even think or plan her next day.

But the one thing she loves doing is watching her saas-bahu soaps on TV. So while she makes her kids study she watches the soaps at night (in mute mode — she does not feel worthy enough to give herself that time. It's almost as if she feels guilty if she is doing anything for herself. She wants to be an ideal mom, ideal wife and homemaker!)

Modifications

Now, Priya is probably doing a great job taking care of her kids and the house. But given a choice, this is not the kind of life she wanted. Although she loves her kids and husband, she had never thought her life would be 'devoted' only to them, and that she would have to compromise on things that she would like to do.

So if Priya starts making simple changes in her daily routine, and starts taking care of her food to begin with, she will have the energy to cope with her daily chores. As her body gets the nourishment it needs, she will feel calmer and not be as stressed as she feels right now.

She can modify her diet as follows:

Meal 1 (7.00 a.m., on rising, within 10 mins): Soaked almonds + walnuts

Meal 2 (8.30 a.m.): Paratha or koki (finally she would eat her Sindhi breakfast, guilt-free)

Meal 3 (10.30 a.m.): Fruit

Meal 4 (11.30 a.m. post workout): Protein shake + boiled potato

Meal 5 (1.00 p.m.): Rice + rajma or channa + sabzi

Meal 6 (3.00 p.m.): Olives (she loves olives, but didn't ever dare to have them)

Meal 7 (5.00 p.m.): Paneer roll (she absolutely looked forward to this meal)

Meal 8 (7.00 p.m.) : Fresh fruit (this was her kids' study time, so she needed steady energy)

Meal 9 (8.30 p.m.): Roti + sabzi

Along with these changes in her diet, she also started working out regularly.

She was asked to take a B6 supplement (to calm her nerves), antioxidants Vitamin C and E, Omega-3 (to improve nutrient delivery to her cells) and calcium so that her body would have the adequate amounts of these essential nutrients to function efficiently.

Also, as she started eating like this, she had a calm and rested sleep (earlier she was too stressed to sleep well) and woke up fresh every morning.

Her children's exams did not stress her out anymore!

As she started eating right, her kids also started to eat like her. Their junk food (biscuits, chips, dessert) were relegated to a once-a-week treat on the weekend, which Priya also indulged in along with them.

Usha Rao is a thirty-three-year-old teacher who runs her own school.

She has been to various dieticians in the past, and because she put on weight every time she got 'off' the diet, she hardly eats anything now, basically surviving on five-six cups of tea a day.

She has constant headaches and takes a painkiller every day and is also exhausted with work and other responsibilities by the end of the day. She is a well-read and motivated teacher, and believes that the headache is simply an occupational hazard and by-product of constantly being around children. She loves being around kids and finds teaching rewarding, but wishes that it didn't come with headaches and the feeling of not being able to keep up with her students' energy levels.

Three-day diet recall

Time	Food/ Drink	Activity Recall	Workout
Day 1			
5.30 – 6.00 a.m.	2-3 cups tea	Woke up	
6.00 – 7.30 a.m.		Got ready, helped my daughter get ready for school	
8.00 a.m.	5 almonds	Dropped my daughter to school and left for the gym	
8.30 – 10.00 a.m.			20 minutes running on treadmill — speed 7.5 20 minutes walk — speed 6 30 minutes cross trainer (level 5-6)
10.30 a.m.		Took a shower and got ready for work	

10.45 a.m. – 2.00 p.m.		Worked on the computer	
1.00 p.m.	1 Mysore masala dosa		
2.00 – 3.00 p.m.		Picked up my daughter from school and dropped her home	
3.00 p.m.	Tea	Left for work	
4.30 p.m.	Tea		
6.00 p.m.	Tea		
7.30 p.m.		Took my daughter swimming	Walked
9.00 p.m.	Vegetable + dal		
9.30 p.m.		Watched TV and then crashed	
Day 2			
5.30 – 6.00 a.m.	1 cup tea	Woke up	
6.00 – 7.30 a.m.		Got ready, helped my daughter to get ready	
8.00 a.m.	5 almonds	Dropped her to school and left for the gym	
8.30 – 10.00 a.m.			20 minutes running 25 minutes walking
10.30 a.m.		Get ready and left for work	
10.45 a.m. – 2.00 p.m.		Worked on computer	
11.00 a.m.	Tea		
12.00 p.m.	Tea		
1.00 p.m.	Tea		
1.30 p.m.	1 cup brown rice, dal, sabzi, curd		
2.00 – 3.00 p.m.		Picked up my daughter from school and dropped her home	

3.00 – 6.00 p.m.		Worked on computer, in class	
7.00 p.m.	1 cup tea and 2 khakra	Played with daughter, gave her dinner	
9.00 p.m.	Roti-sabzi	TV	
Day 3 (Holiday)			
6.30 a.m.	2 cups tea	Woke up	
8.00 a.m.		Showered and got ready	
9.00 a.m.	1 slice of brown bread + 1 egg white omelette		
9.30 a.m.		Left for daughter's class	
1.30 p.m.	Lunch out	Back from class	
3.30 – 5.00 p.m.		Afternoon nap	
5.00 p.m.	2 cups tea	In bed, watching TV	
10.00 p.m.	1 roti + sabzi and a small bowl of curd		

Evaluation of the recall

Because Usha put on weight in the past after going 'off' a diet, she does not eat much through the day, thinking that not eating will help her lose weight. However, instead of having tea nearly five-six times a day, if she eats food that will provide her body with the nutrients it needs, she will not have headaches, nor will she feel fatigued at the end of the day. Plus, there's the added benefit of losing fat (she is basically having tea to mask her appetite and to go without food for as long as possible).

Usha has a very long day. She wakes up early, exercises, goes to work and takes care of her daughter, but she is so caught up with work she is unaware of what she needs to provide her body with and at what time of the day. When you eat so little and when you have such long gaps between your meals, the body learns to store fat.

Modifications

If she eats well, giving her body the right nutrients at the right time, and reduces her intake of tea, Usha will start feeling more energetic, healthier, and she will not have headaches.

She can modify her diet as follows:

Meal 1 (6.00 a.m.): Handful of dry fruit

Meal 2 (7.30 a.m.): Banana

Meal 3 (9.30 a.m., post workout): Fruit + protein shake

Meal 4 (10.30 a.m.): Fresh homemade breakfast (poha/upma/just about anything that's fresh and hot from the kitchen)

Meal 5 (12.30 p.m.): Coconut water + malai (she loves it but never had it thinking it was fattening)

Meal 6 (1.30 p.m.): Roti + sabzi + dal (easy for her as she was lucky enough to have access to fresh home-cooked food)

Meal 7 (3.30 p.m.): Handful of peanuts (convenient to have in between classes)

Meal 8 (5.30 p.m.): Soya milk

Meal 9 (7.30 p.m.): Fruit (easy to have while she is out of the house with her daughter for her swimming class)

Meal 9 (8.30 p.m.): Paneer sabzi + roti or chicken + sabzi + roti

Instead of tea, she should drink much more water throughout the day, which will help keep her vocal cords lubricated and ease the stress on her voice box. ☺

Usha followed this eating pattern for two weeks and her diet was changed regularly. She was also taking B-complex, vitamins C and E, flaxseed and calcium supplements.

Within a week of eating right, she realised that her craving for tea was almost gone and she didn't need a painkiller anymore for her headaches. For her, this was nothing short of a miracle; for me, it's a natural consequence of stable blood sugars.

Now to function efficiently through the day, we need to ensure that our blood glucose levels remain at an optimum. This can only be achieved by eating the right food at regular intervals.

Tea is only a stimulant and therefore gives you that kick to keep you going. But what you are actually doing by having tea each time you are hungry is suppressing your appetite, and because your body is nutrient-deficient you end up feeling tired and fatigued by the end of the day.

As soon as Usha started eating as per her body's requirements, her cells received the nutrition as required and so she didn't feel low on energy — therefore, she did not feel the need for tea. She was able to keep up with her kids and felt as energetic as them!

Usha was very lucky to have her husband's support while she was on the diet as they both did it together. They kept motivating one another and if one slipped-up, the other would push the partner back on track. This really added a new dimension to her marriage!

Acknowledgements

These are just some of the people I would like to thank sincerely and profusely because in more ways than one they have made this book happen. I know this can never really do full justice, but here goes…

- My readers for debating, discussing, adapting and adopting my writing to their eating and living in such a wholesome manner that I can't but feel deep gratitude for this generosity and kindness. Thanks for making me a part of your life, truly … thanks :)

- To all the health professionals, yoga teachers, doctors, trainers, physios whom I have worked with for sharing their stories of the 'tamasha', for choosing to handle health with the integrity it deserves and for spreading awareness on weight loss/BMI/ideal weight, etc. being outdated concepts and misleading measures of health and fitness.

- My clients for being the most driven, dedicated and disciplined species on earth, for always eating sensibly and on time and for always letting me walk away with the entire credit for their hardcore efforts.

- My friend Mahesha of Japro Engineering for sharing the process of making fatty acids and extracting oil in so much detail that I really had a hard time putting all of that in a box.

- My sister Ankita, for nobody on earth is as sharp, witty, beautiful and brave as she is. And my three-year-old nephew Sunay for his ability to clearly know what he wants to do, eat, read, etc. E.g. any book without pictures is not worth reading and that includes mine.

- My parents, especially my mom for translating this book into Marathi, with a focus, I must confess, that puts the writer in me to shame.

- My team of nutritionists, Tejal, Puujaa, Jhanvi, for compiling my data and for all the masala chai evenings in office.

- Bebo, for the straight-from-the-heart handwritten note, all in between globe-trotting and twenty-hour workdays.

- My beautiful editor Deepthi, for restoring my faith in the humane side of editors and for being so beautifully patient.

- And of course GP, for being man enough to keep his feminine side alive, for 'Connect with Himalaya', for painstakingly reading and re-reading my writing and for making this book what it is.

Rujuta Diwekar works out of Mumbai, practises yoga in Rishikesh, ideates in Uttarkashi and treks in the rest of the Indian Himalaya. Winner of the Nutrition Award 2010 from Asian Institute of Gastroenterology, she is amongst the most qualified and sought-after practitioners in India today and the only nutritionist to have accreditation from Sports Dietitians, Australia. Her first book sold more than two lakh copies in four languages and is still in national best-seller lists, more than a hundred weeks after its debut.

In the plethora of diet fads and fears, Rujuta's voice rings loud and clear, urging us to use our common sense and un-complicate the act of eating. With over a decade of experience working with people from all walks of life, including Kareena Kapoor, Anil Ambani, Preity Zinta, Karishma Kapoor, Saif Ali Khan and Konkona Sen Sharma, she has fine-tuned her methods to the real issues facing urban Indians.

A bit more:

Rujuta regularly practices and studies the Iyengar tradition of yoga and has also completed Sadhna Intensive and teacher training courses from Sivananda Yog Vedanta academy.

She is actively involved in various farming practices at her family-owned farm in Sonave, just outside Mumbai.

A much sought-after speaker, she has conducted workshops for corporates, clubs, fundraisers, schools, etc in India and abroad.